Surviving and Thriving in Midwifery

T0327691

Surviving and Thriving in Midwifery

Written by

Sally Pezaro

Karen Maher

WILEY Blackwell

This edition first published 2025
© 2025 John Wiley & Sons Ltd

All rights reserved, including rights for text and data mining and training of artificial technologies or similar technologies. No part of this publication may be reproduced, stored in a retrieval system, or transmitted, in any form or by any means, electronic, mechanical, photocopying, recording or otherwise, except as permitted by law. Advice on how to obtain permission to reuse material from this title is available at http://www.wiley.com/go/permissions.

The right of Sally Pezaro and Karen Maher to be identified as the authors of the editorial material in this work has been asserted in accordance with law.

Registered Office(s)
John Wiley & Sons, Inc., 111 River Street, Hoboken, NJ 07030, USA
John Wiley & Sons Ltd, New Era House, 8 Oldlands Way, Bognor Regis, West Sussex, PO22 9NQ, UK

For details of our global editorial offices, customer services, and more information about Wiley products visit us at www.wiley.com.

The manufacturer's authorized representative according to the EU General Product Safety Regulation is Wiley-VCH GmbH, Boschstr. 12, 69469 Weinheim, Germany, e-mail: Product_Safety@wiley.com.

Wiley also publishes its books in a variety of electronic formats and by print-on-demand. Some content that appears in standard print versions of this book may not be available in other formats.

Trademarks: Wiley and the Wiley logo are trademarks or registered trademarks of John Wiley & Sons, Inc. and/or its affiliates in the United States and other countries and may not be used without written permission. All other trademarks are the property of their respective owners. John Wiley & Sons, Inc. is not associated with any product or vendor mentioned in this book.

Limit of Liability/Disclaimer of Warranty
The contents of this work are intended to further general scientific research, understanding, and discussion only and are not intended and should not be relied upon as recommending or promoting scientific method, diagnosis, or treatment by physicians for any particular patient. In view of ongoing research, equipment modifications, changes in governmental regulations, and the constant flow of information relating to the use of medicines, equipment, and devices, the reader is urged to review and evaluate the information provided in the package insert or instructions for each medicine, equipment, or device for, among other things, any changes in the instructions or indication of usage and for added warnings and precautions. While the publisher and authors have used their best efforts in preparing this work, they make no representations or warranties with respect to the accuracy or completeness of the contents of this work and specifically disclaim all warranties, including without limitation any implied warranties of merchantability or fitness for a particular purpose. No warranty may be created or extended by sales representatives, written sales materials or promotional statements for this work. This work is sold with the understanding that the publisher is not engaged in rendering professional services. The advice and strategies contained herein may not be suitable for your situation. You should consult with a specialist where appropriate. The fact that an organization, website, or product is referred to in this work as a citation and/or potential source of further information does not mean that the publisher and authors endorse the information or services the organization, website, or product may provide or recommendations it may make. Further, readers should be aware that websites listed in this work may have changed or disappeared between when this work was written and when it is read. Neither the publisher nor authors shall be liable for any loss of profit or any other commercial damages, including but not limited to special, incidental, consequential, or other damages.

Library of Congress Cataloging-in-Publication Data Applied for
Paperback ISBN: 9781119881001

Cover Design: Wiley
Cover Images: © Fly View Productions/Getty Images, © bibikoff/Getty Images, © Iwaria Inc./UnSplash

Set in 10.5/13pt STIXTwoText by Straive, Pondicherry, India

Contents

List of Contributors

Mariama Lilei Feika, MSc, BSc (Hons) RN, RM
Director of Nursing & Midwifery
Al Khor Hospital – Hamad Medical Corporation
Qatar

Sadie Geraghty, RM, PhD
National Head of Discipline (Midwifery)
National School of Nursing & Midwifery
Faculty of Medicine, Nursing, Midwifery and Health Sciences
The University of Notre Dame Australia

Fiona Gibb, MRes, PgCert HELT, BM, RM, SFHEA
Director, Professional Midwifery
Royal College of Midwives
London, UK

Pandora Hardtman, DNP, CNM, RN, FACNM, FAAN
Johns Hopkins Program for International Education in Gynecology and Obstetrics
Johns Hopkins University
Baltimore, MD, USA

Inderjeet Kaur, Msc
Director of Midwifery Services
Fernandez Foundation
Hyderabad, Telangana, India

Harriet Nayiga, BScM
Founding director
Midwife-led Community Transformation (MILCOT)
Kampala, Central Region
Uganda

Ruth Oshikanlu, MBE, QN, FiHV FRCN, FRSA, PhD
MBE Queen's Nurse, Fellow of The Royal College of Nursing, Fellow of The Royal Society for Public Health; Independent Midwife, Health Visitor and Pregnancy Mindset Expert; CEO Goal Mind
London, UK

John Pendleton, PhD
University of Northampton
Waterside Campus, University Drive, Northampton, UK

Dr Jan Smith, PhD
Chartered Psychologist, Founder
Healthy You Ltd & MindYourself
Huddersfield, UK

Mary E. Fissell, PhD
Inaugural J. Mario Molina Professor in the History of Medicine,
Department of the History of Medicine,
Johns Hopkins University

Amanda Burleigh, RGN, RN, BSc
Midwifery Consultant

Author Contact Details and Biographies

Dr Sally Pezaro
School of Nursing, Midwifery and Health, Coventry University,
Priory Street, Coventry, CV1 5FB
E-mail: sally.pezaro@coventry.ac.uk

Dr Sally Pezaro is a registered Midwife, an Assistant Professor at Coventry University in the UK, an adjunct Associate Professor at the University of Notre Dame in Australia, a Fellow of the Royal College of Midwives (FRCM) and an editorial board member of Evidence Based Midwifery, MIDIRS and the International Journal of Childbirth. She is also a regulatory panellist, Senior Fellow of the Higher Education Academy (SFHEA), an Invited member of the Ehlers-Danlos Society's International Consortium and lead midwife for www.hEDSTogether.com. Dr Pezaro has clinical midwifery experience working in the United Kingdom, the Gambia and Ethiopia. Reflecting on her own experiences, Dr Pezaro ensures that her work, now in research and academia remains challenge led.

The Ehlers-Danlos Society bestowed Dr Pezaro with the 'Outstanding Consortium Member of the Year' award in 2022. In 2021, Dr Pezaro also won a 'Midwives Award' from the Iolanthe Midwifery Trust and a 'Partnership Working' award from the Royal College of Midwives. In 2019, Dr Pezaro was honoured with a first prize award from the Royal Society of Medicine in 'Leading and inspiring excellence in maternity care' and was also the first runner-up for the British Journal of Midwifery's 'Midwife of the Year' 2019.

The overriding vision for Dr Pezaro's ongoing work is to secure psychologically safe professional journeys and excellence in healthcare. Follow her on social media @SallyPezaro

Dr Karen Maher
Department of Work and Organisation, Aston Business School,
Aston University, Aston Triangle, Birmingham, B4 7ET
E-mail: k.maher1@aston.ac.uk

Karen is a Chartered Psychologist and Lecturer at Aston Business School whose work specialises in Occupational Health and Work Well-being. She completed her PhD in Work Psychology at Loughborough University in 2018, which focused on employee well-being and shift working in the Fire and Rescue Service. Prior to moving to Academia, Karen was a Health, Fitness and Well-being practitioner with expertise in GP Exercise Referral, exercise rehabilitation and weight management. Previous roles included Health and Well-being Advisor within the Fire Service, responsible for behaviour change programmes for fitness, stress and weight/disease management for operational and support staff using one-to-one coaching and group programmes. Her research is currently centred on behaviour change within the workplace to improve the safety and health of workers with projects exploring maladaptive coping techniques in the workplace (substance use, counterproductive work behaviours), and adherence to safety policies and procedures. Karen was Chair of the Organisational Psychology Special Interest Group at the British Academy of Management from 2019 to 2022.

Foreword

When I was given the title of this book, I couldn't help but smile at the catchphrase survive and thrive. Survive and thrive, some days it feels like we hang on by our fingertips to sanity, oftentimes fuelled by lack of sleep, an overabundance of work, rage, hope and despair and joy in equal measure. We are midwives!

Survive and Thrive was an alliance of government, professional health association, private sector and non-profit partners working with country governments and health professionals to improve health outcomes for mothers, newborns and children through clinical training, systems strengthening and policy advocacy funded by the United States Agency for International Development. Survive and Thrive then went on to become Survive, Thrive and Transform impacting millions of lives over the years of the project and beyond.

Though the programme has ended I must say that true words have never been spoken, interestingly, the campaign also dealt with addressing shortfalls in maternal health and child healthcare, sounds like this was written by and for midwives, doesn't it?

The key to survival in midwifery is truly about just that ability to adapt, evolve and grow.

More than twenty-five years later, I can say although the sayings may sound tried and true that is exactly true. When I look at my career there is pretty much no aspect of women's sexual reproductive health that I have not tried on for size and I am grateful that we have so many competencies from which to choose.

How we survive doesn't have to look like how anybody else does it, as we are all rooted and grounded in the philosophy of midwifery which says and reminds us that we have a grounding and are rooted in the normal biological and psychosocial definitions of reproductive health across the lifespan. Sometimes surviving and thriving is about letting go. Letting go of myself and images of what it should be like. I'll never forget a particular couple that I worked with. This couple was special to me in that I was working in the expanded scope of midwifery practice and working with couples through artificial insemination to become parents. Needless to say, we succeeded and had a series of amazing antenatal visits and close to three years had gone by. By this time, I have been working intensively with this particular family for over two years. The pregnancy progressed while the couple were glowing. They were financially comfortable, supportive family all around them, things couldn't be better. And then one day she walked in at 36 weeks for her normal routine visit, and we could not find foetal heart tones. I was devastated and ran to get the sonogram machine from the next-door. The sonogram machine confirmed my worst fears which I refused to believe because these things just don't happen. Within the hour the radiographer confirmed our worst fears the much-loved little boy had passed on to his next journey before ever taking a breath in this realm. The difficult decision was to move forward with an immediate induction of labour which turned into a long two-day process. The mother who had previously planned for an epidural now opted to have an unmedicated birth. Though it seemed simple, it was somehow complicated by the fact that most of the new nurses were uncomfortable with supporting an unmedicated mother. And so, I stayed by her bedside until this beautiful baby boy was born into our arms three days later. We cried together. Bereavement boxes, handprints, footprints and little locks of hair cut to be cherished. And the mother sat in the chair and rocked, and I sat on the couch and cried, and we all cried together. Forget the stiff upper lip; I could not hold it together. I did not think that I could go on, we had come so far together and now this. I wanted to quit midwifery altogether. The rollercoaster of emotions was just too much and so we grieved together, we got through and we stayed connected for years thereafter, even after I had changed jobs. Thus, I survived and thrived in a new environment leaving fertility care behind and my care was transformed by adversity.

One of my greatest concerns, like many others, is how to maintain the midwifery workforce of the current and into the future. We can all attest to the trends of textbooks that are being written as we continue to advance the evidence behind midwifery practice. Textbooks that provide the core of our practice. However, sadly lacking are the stories. Much of what we hear about our profession is shaped by a media that does not always understand us and really is made to sell different kinds of stories that are dramatic, feeding the public adrenaline rush. There are also the novels that romanticise reality often serving to paint a false paradigm of the day in and day out. This has left a gap. A gap in the narrative, and this is truly where I feel the beauty of this particular book can shine through. There will be good days and there will be bad days, there is simply no getting around that. This is why we need more of these kinds of books to add to our own mythology of midwifery. It is the stories of how to move on in trying times, the learning from the Aunties, the elders and the sisters to teach, to inspire and to keep us going.

Our stories are our lessons to the next generation. I am often asked how have you made it for so long? How did you do that. Well, the answer is simply survive, thrive and transform, harking back to the title of this book. With a solid basic foundation, we can do anything. Midwives can and must do everything if we are truly to change the face of maternal health nationally and globally. Not just sticking to the viewpoint from the perineum, but truly evolving into other spaces. The beauty of this book is that through a narrative tale, it gives us a pathway by which we may evolve into other spaces that we may not have been previously shown.

Thriving in midwifery is also about finding joy in the little things. It's not just chocolates and flowers and thank you's, but the gentle smile, the gentle touch. It's the ability to find a midwife friend who gets it even if she is half away around the world and you don't talk to her every day. On the days you can't find that friend, pick up this book. Pick up this book and know that you are part of a vital profession with a legacy of strength. Midwifery is ancient as wisdom, modern as time.

Pandora Hardtman, DNP, CNM, RN, FACNM, FAAN
Chief Nursing and Midwifery Officer
Johns Hopkins Program for International Education
in Gynaecology and Obstetrics (Jhpiego)

Preface

I have wanted to become a midwife ever since my sibling came into the world and I saw what the awesome human body could do. I have practised as a midwife in the United Kingdom, The Gambia and Ethiopia. Yet it has been over a decade now since I almost did not survive midwifery. After a turbulent time with ill health and incivility, I went where I was celebrated and could grow from my experiences. Now each day, the research and academic work I do in midwifery is me working not just to survive like I did back then, but to thrive.

I wanted to share my personal story throughout this book in the hope that it may give light and solidarity to other midwives in darkness, or those who are unsure how to maximise their potential.

> *When we deny our stories, they define us. When we own our stories, we get to write a brave new ending.*
>
> – Brené Brown

I am a Tall Poppy. Yet making sense of the world around me does not come easy, and I must work hard to push to new levels of understanding every day. In this book, I share what I have learnt over the years in the hope that it will enable other midwives not just to survive but thrive in the profession more easily than I have. Nevertheless, success requires more than just one person. As such, this book draws from several diverse voices in midwifery to bring surviving and thriving in the profession to life. I also draw upon the wisdom of my dear friend, colleague and co-author Dr Karen Maher in this book, to gain perspective from the field of occupational psychology.

This book is the gift I want to give to my earlier self.

KAREN

Over the years, I have reflected on why some work leaves me energised and other work leaves me drained and came to the realisation that, if what I was being asked to do did not align with my core values, over time it would deplete me. The longer this goes on the more likely I am to feel symptoms of stress and strain. My core value is about supporting people to navigate challenges, both internal and external, to become the best versions of themselves, which was why I was so happy to be invited to be part of this book.

Part of becoming the best person we can be is about looking inwards; pick up any self-help book or wellness manual and it pretty much centres around the individual and how they can change. However, helping people become the best version of themselves sometimes involves challenging the system, the structural issues that create barriers to thriving. This is very much the way Sally and I have approached this book, providing the tools to be able to help you navigate the system you are working in whilst calling out those things that need to change and how you can be part of that.

Prior to becoming an academic, I worked in occupational health with frontline workers in the emergency services and noticed the toll their work has on their well-being and their families. Whilst still working in occupational health, I retrained as a psychologist as it was the psychological part of my job that fascinated me. However, my experience working in practice still shapes the research and psychological work I hold dear, and I strive to support those who carry out a critical role in society. I very much take an evidence-based approach to address practical issues and want my research to have a societal purpose. For me, academic work is only useful if it makes a difference to those we include in research, rather than being lost in an academic journal for all eternity. That involves sharing our knowledge in ways just like this book, where it will be read by exactly the people who may benefit.

It is important to add that I am not a midwife so my voice may feel different as you navigate the book, but hopefully you can see the value in bringing a psychological perspective to the world of midwifery.

We are on this planet for such a short time so let's do what we can to thrive and flourish!

Acknowledgements

Writing this book has been a culmination of conversations and collaborations engaged in by both of us over the course of our careers. Firstly, we would like to give heartfelt thanks to the midwives across the globe who have contributed their comments and thoughts for inclusion in the book. For ethical reasons we have kept these contributions anonymous but we value the richness these voices bring to the concepts under discussion in each of the chapters. We are also grateful to all the colleagues and contributors (too many to mention but each are credited alongside their contributions with mutual agreement) who have inspired the direction of this book along with the themes and sections within it.

Throughout this book, we use many retrospective examples to outline the concepts and ideas we explore. As such, we must also express gratitude to those who shared their examples and acknowledge the vulnerability and openness that allows for the learning to happen from these experiences.

We are also inspired by the many midwives and student midwives who demonstrate passion and enthusiasm for their profession, and the desire and determination to survive and thrive despite adversity every day. This book is predominantly written for you.

Lastly, we understand that our lived experience has shaped our writing of this book and acknowledge the privilege it brings to our experience of midwifery, academia and navigating the world. Through this position we seek to challenge injustice and promote equality, diversity and inclusion through collaboration and public acts of advocacy. These values have guided our exploration of topics within the book. We may not always get it right, but we remain committed to learning how we can best elevate the voices of others.

List of Figures

List of Tables

CHAPTER 1

Introduction

INTRO TO CHAPTER

The Lancet Series on midwifery published in 2014 outlined the specific and vital role of midwives in the provision of high-quality perinatal and newborn health and care around the world (ten Hoope-Bender and Renfrew 2014). Nevertheless, there are global reports of midwifery workforce shortages linked to recruitment and retention issues. Moreover, the midwives currently in post are not always empowered to practise in the way they need or want to. Furthermore, some have limited autonomy and others require upskilling. These global challenges may not be solved in one book. Yet this book is needed to offer midwives a personalised toolkit from which to draw when they themselves need to survive and thrive in the face of challenges.

Due to their role in public health and reproductive services, empowered midwives also have the potential to contribute towards achieving the world's sustainable development goals (United Nations 2015). Yet we have highlighted how midwifery is often undervalued and underserved (Pezaro et al. 2022b). Where conventionally, professions are granted autonomy and social recognition for the services they provide, midwifery often lacks such status.

Nursing in comparison with midwifery has a robust history with widely revered figures, such as Clara Barton and Florence Nightingale. Although such figures have complex historical legacies, crucially those complexities derive from real life, serving to ground the identity of nursing. Thus, historical and reflective narratives of midwifery might similarly serve to ground the contemporary identity of midwifery.

Midwifery can be conflated with other professions (e.g. nursing), which challenges the creation of a distinctive professional identity and status. For midwives to be fully valued and play a crucial role in reducing global maternal and neonatal deaths, we argue their professional identity must be firmly instantiated.

Surviving and Thriving in Midwifery, First Edition. Sally Pezaro and Karen Maher.
© 2025 John Wiley & Sons Ltd. Published 2025 by John Wiley & Sons Ltd.

History can tell us who we are, where we come from, and thus may guide us as to where we are going. Therefore, we start this book by introducing a historical narrative of midwifery, written by Professor Mary Fissell, as much of what is available on the history of midwifery is rooted in mythic or fictional characters such as Agnodike or Sairey Gamp. We then give an overview of the challenges faced within contemporary midwifery and explain what to expect from this book overall. As you read the historical narrative below, reflect on what we can learn about ourselves as midwives in terms of where we come from, who we are and where we may be going in future.

You may notice gender and culture wars apparent in this historical narrative, dressed up as Man versus Woman. It is important to reflect on how our history has shaped us as a profession, but at the same time avoid judging the past by present standards and ideals. We recognise the challenges midwifery faces in relation to gender inequalities and will address some of these issues later in the book. For now, we request, with whichever gender you identify (or not), you read the following with only a curiosity for how midwifery of the past was perceived.

CIRCUMSTANCES, WHICH NO MAN CAN BE A JUDGE OF: SARAH STONE AND THE IMPROVEMENT OF MIDWIFERY

Sarah Stone (c. 1680–1737) was really tired. The early eighteenth-century Somerset midwife had travelled 10 miles on horseback over terrible roads to support a soap-boiler's wife in childbirth, whose usual midwife could not be found. On the way there, a man ran up to her, and asked if they had seen another midwife, who, it turned out, was a further 8 miles away. After supporting the soap-boiler's wife to birth her baby, Stone called in at the other woman's house and was told that they had found another midwife and the baby would be born in the quarter of an hour. So, Stone rode home. But it was not to be. Five hours later, the second husband came to Stone and begged her to return, saying her women feared the baby would never be born.

After her services had been refused earlier, she had to travel back to the same house on the same bad road. Once there, Stone demonstrated to her skills, 'as soon as I Touched her, I was sensible of the reason of this poor Woman's being kept so long in distress' (Stone 1737, p. 71). Her hands knew what was the matter; 'touching' was a newly coined technical term for manual examination (Giffard 1734, pp. 26, 44, 50, 53). Stone aided the woman to give birth quickly and concluded the case by saying 'for 'tis an undoubted rule, If Pains do no good, they do a great deal of harm' (Stone 1737, p. 73). Repeatedly, Stone abstracted such general rules from her daily practice, creating new knowledge and disseminating it in print. She wrote movingly about the pains birthing women suffered and criticised other midwives whose incompetence left women labouring for longer than necessary.

Stone's history contrasts with the narratives historians often tell about eighteenth-century English midwifery (Wilson 1995). For it was in Stone's own lifetime that men began to assist with the birth of babies in England. The period is often portrayed as a turf battle between men, armed with the new technology of obstetrical forceps, and women who had long been the primary carers for pregnant and parturient women. Casting the eighteenth century in this way has caused us to overlook the work midwives did to make births safer; Stone is an excellent example of such pioneering work. In this essay, I will show how Stone sought to improve the practice of midwifery, and put her work in the larger context of enlightenment midwifery in Europe (Grundy 1995; Marland 1993).

We know about Stone's life and practice because she published a book of her cases in 1737; she was only the second midwife to publish in English. She was born around 1680, and married Samuel Stone in 1700; two of their children were baptised in the same Bridgwater parish over the next few years. Stone trained with her mother, who was a noted local midwife, and then served as her mother's deputy for six years, basically in joint practice. Her mother died in 1708, and Stone embarked upon a solo practice (*Bridgewater St Mary's Parish Records;* 1682–1714). One of her biggest constraints was that noted above: the roads were terrible. Over the course of her career, Stone moved to Taunton, then Bristol, and finally London, where she died not long after the publication of her book. Her daughter, trained by Stone, worked in Bristol as a midwife.

Stone worked both as a regular midwife, with a list of clients who booked her in advance for their births, and as a consultant midwife, called in when things went wrong, as in the case described above (Woods and Galley 2014). Her caseload was staggering; she claims to have assisted as many as 300 births a year when she was in Somerset. Even half that number is astonishing, and indicates that much of her work was consultant, summoned in a crisis, possibly seeing a client for only a few hours. Her book was likely written in part as advertising when she moved to London. By then Samuel was dead, and she would have wanted to attract customers in the metropolis.

While self-promotion may have been a factor, Stone's goal was to improve the standards of midwifery. She dedicated her book to the Queen, whom she described as 'the Nursing-mother' of the nation; the book was intended to 'prove instructive' to female midwives, especially rural and lower-class ones (Stone 1737, pp. vi, vii). By the 1730s, Stone had encountered the new breed of male midwife, and she was scathing about them, saying 'that almost every young Man, who has served his Apprenticeship to a Barber-Surgeon, immediately sets up for a Man-Midwife' (Stone 1737, p. xi). She repeatedly characterised man-midwives as boyish and ignorant (Stone 1737, p. xiv). While Stone had attended anatomical dissections, she did not consider such training to be sufficient, 'For dissecting the Dead, and being just and tender to the Living, are vastly different' (Stone 1737, p. xiv). She staked a claim to women's particular expertise in midwifery, 'there is a tender regard one Woman bears to another, and a natural Sympathy in those that have gone thro' the Pangs of Childbearing'. Men lacked understanding because they had not given birth; those were 'circumstances, which no man can be a judge of' (Stone 1737, pp. xiv–xv). A combination of empathy and experience made a judicious midwife.

However, Stone was also very critical of female midwives who did not know enough to be skilled practitioners. In a difficult situation with a woman who had been in labour for four days already, Stone argued with the midwife who had been attending the woman. 'I asked her Midwife the reason, Why she did not deliver her? She told me, Because God's time was not come: (a common saying amongst illiterate unskilful Midwives)' Stone retorted dryly, 'that it appeared to me to be God's time then'. Stone described the mother as 'to the eye of Reason, very near death', but she managed to save her life (Stone 1737, pp. 44–45).

Another case demonstrated similar failings in rural midwifery care. A woman in Bishop's Lydeard went into labour on a Friday and on Saturday she birthed a child. When the midwife went to deliver the afterbirth, she found that there were twins. The midwife assured the mother that 'when the other Apple was ripe it would also fall'. Stone commented 'O ignorance!'. On Sunday the husband sent for Stone, fearing his wife would not live. She told the story with great drama, 'we rode as fast as possible, and 'twas but 5 miles from Taunton, yet we had two messengers sent after us for expedition, for all her Women thought her dying' (Stone 1737, p. 66). Stone managed to assist in the birth of the second child after an hour and a half of hard work. The moral pointed to the skill and knowledge needed in a midwife, 'For 'tis certain, if the Midwife understands her business as she ought, she might bring the second child soon after the first: for generally in the birth of twins, when the first is born the other should be brought by Art'. Stone added that she never put a woman 'to any more than ten- or fifteen-minutes pain after I had delivered her of the first child' (Stone 1737, p. 68). Stone declared that this case rested upon a basic fact that ought to be known by all midwives: when one twin was born naturally, skill and manipulation were needed to deliver the second one.

In addition to elucidating these kinds of fundamental rules, Stone also modelled knowledge-making for her midwife readers. She recorded exceptional cases, problems that might only happen to a midwife once in her career. Many of Stone's colleagues encountered very few difficult births because they had relatively low caseloads, assisting in the birth of perhaps 20 babies a year, with perhaps a single birth per year presenting difficulties (Wilson 1995, p. 33). Stone, with her mix of regular and consultant midwifery, saw as many or more difficult births in a year than some midwives saw in their entire career.

A tragic birth in Taunton models for Stone's readers how to make knowledge from an exceptional case. Stone was called late at night to see a wool comber's wife. The woman had gone into labour around noon, called her midwife, and been delivered standing up. The woman's midwife, described by Stone, as 'a feeble ancient woman', was unable to deliver the placenta. The navel-string (what we'd call the 'umbilical cord') broke close to the placenta, and the mother bled copiously (Stone 1737, p. 54). By the time Stone arrived, the mother was past recovery. Stone tried to imagine what had happened and deduced that it was a combination of a very short navel-string, the standing posture which accelerated labour and the weakness of the midwife who did not support the child, whose weight, combined with the too-short cord, initiated the bleeding. Up till this point, the reader is led to believe that this is a perfect storm caused by the rare intersection of three different factors.

But Stone continued this case by describing how three or four years later, she attended a gentlewoman whom she had assisted in childbirth several times before. When the infant could not be birthed, she remembered this earlier case and found that the cord was pulled tight. She kept a tight hold on the cord, allowed the baby to birth, and then, in under seven minutes, the placenta. Both mother and child did well. Stone thus modelled for the reader how to draw upon previous experience to make a working hypothesis in a difficult case, test the hypothesis with her hands (feeling the navel-string strained), and act upon the tested hypothesis. She noted a general rule to be abstracted from these two cases, namely that women should give birth in bed, rather than standing, and that a midwife should be one of 'judgement and activity', that is both wise and able to act decisively (Stone 1737, p. 58).

Stone was exceptional in English midwifery; her cases are written in almost novelistic detail and give us vivid pictures of her practice. We simply do not know how many other highly skilled consultant midwives were practising in eighteenth-century England. However, Stone's plan to improve the standards of midwifery by combatting ignorance was echoed by subsequent English midwives such as Elizabeth Nihell and Martha Mears, who published their own books to educate midwives (Cody 2005). Further afield, other midwives similarly sought to improve standards. Justine Siegemund (1636–1706) published a midwifery guide in the form of a dialogue between herself and one of her pupils; it included a novel method for a shoulder delivery. At her funeral, it was said that she had assisted in the births of almost 6200 babies over the course of her career (Tatlock 2005). In France, Angélique Marguerite Le Boursier du Coudray (c. 1712–1794) developed a new programme for training provincial midwives using life-sized obstetrical models to demonstrate a wide variety of presentations. Louis XV commissioned her to take her teaching programme to various cities and towns. From 1760–1783 she trained 4000 students and her students taught another 6000 (Gelbart 1998).

Such enlightenment-era midwives were actively teaching and improving practice. Narratives that emphasise conflict between male midwives and female ones often describe men as the innovators, and women as left behind. There is an alternate history, however, that reveals a series of women like Sarah Stone, committed to using the medium of print, as well as face-to-face teaching, to help their fellow midwives develop stronger skills and create innovative methods to improve their profession.

Mary E. Fissell, PhD (she/her/hers)
Inaugural J. Mario Molina Professor in the History of Medicine,
Department of the History of Medicine
Johns Hopkins University

CONTEMPORARY MIDWIFERY

Midwives' scope of practice and regulation varies worldwide. Thus contemporarily, the midwifery profession may be somewhat lost in its professional identity, direction and place within the world. Both the art and science of midwifery are balanced to varying degrees around the world too, and so different voices in midwifery can come into conflict. Nevertheless, midwifery needs to remain relevant and contemporary in an ever-evolving world, where the needs of both midwives and people who birth evolve and change. In more recent times, we have had to overcome challenges in embracing digital technology too (Takian et al. 2012). Like Sarah Stone in the previous section, when we know better, we must do better.

Despite the need for us to thrive, throughout the world midwives experience several types of work-related psychological distress. These include both organisational and occupational sources of stress such as workplace bullying, poor organisational cultures, medical errors, traumatic clinical events, critical incidents, occupational stress, workplace suspension, whistleblowing, investigations via professional regulatory bodies and employers, and/or pre-existing mental health conditions (Pezaro et al. 2016). Indeed, whilst midwives have a proud history of speaking out and must continue to engage in whistleblowing where change is required, the consequential bullying, ostracism and blame, combined with structural issues such as insufficient governance and reporting mechanisms are significant (Capper et al. 2024). In recent years, midwives have additionally worked through the global COVID-19 pandemic along with other professional groups in healthcare. The terms moral distress, compassion fatigue, burnout and post-traumatic stress disorder describe the emotional states reported by those working through the COVID-19 pandemic caused by care delivery challenges; insufficient staff and training; challenges with personal protective equipment and frustrations, leading many to consider leaving the profession (Maben et al. 2022). Under the immense pressure and difficult working conditions (e.g. during the COVID-19 pandemic), one's duties can be internalised, and thus relied upon to motivate and sustain staff in the face of personal hardship and oppressive conditions (Anzaldua and Halpern 2021). However, the impact of acting strictly from duty further collapses the space for mental freedom and worsens one's ability to engage with authentic reactions of outrage, fear and grief. In internalising such emotions, we may still be wounded and in need of recovery from all work-related psychological distress associated with being a midwife. Unfortunately, there is a lack of evidence-based interventions available to support both midwives and student midwives in work-related psychological distress (Pezaro et al. 2017), though interventions such as Schwartz Rounds may be useful for some (Ng et al. 2023). In rising from the ashes, a re-imagining of the midwifery profession may now be appropriate as we work to survive and thrive despite adversity in an ever-changing world. In a recent manifesto for change it is suggested that we must prioritise the essential needs of staff; take a systems approach to staff support and share good practice; normalise and anticipate psychological health management; give equal emphasis to psychological and physical harm; nurture compassionate leaders and foster learning over blame cultures (Maben et al. 2023). How might these elements be realised in your area of practice?

Whilst there has been much written about the changing profile of those who birth around the world in terms of demographics, we are also supporting individuals with multiple and long-term conditions more frequently in contemporary midwifery practice. For example, research in the field of childbearing with hypermobile Ehlers Danlos Syndrome (hEDS) and Hypermobility Spectrum Disorders (HSD) has gained much interest as we begin to understand more about the effect of these conditions upon pregnancy and birth (Pezaro et al. 2018b; Pezaro 2021b). These conditions, commonly underdiagnosed are now understood to affect approximately 1 in 20 pregnancies worldwide and have profound and life-threatening consequences in childbearing as they affect connective tissues throughout the body (Pezaro et al. 2020a). Work in this area is gaining traction as we discover more and highlight the needs and care considerations for perinatal staff working with such populations (Pearce et al. 2023a,b). More details on this field of research are available via www.hEDSTogether.com, where toolkits, education and decision-making tools can be freely downloaded for use.

There are also many underserved, minoritised and marginalised groups requiring improved outcomes and care in contemporary perinatal services. Year after year, we see that global majority people (e.g. non-white people) are four to five times more likely to die in childbirth when compared to their white counterparts. Yet it is important to avoid one group acting as 'saviours' for another. Equally, it would be inappropriate to expect any one group to 'fix' the inequalities we observe. For the betterment of midwifery, perinatal services and society it will be important for us all to work towards reducing inequalities in all areas moving forward and embrace diversity. Indeed, whilst the art and science of midwifery remain the same, midwifery work is undertaken in a context where diversity is becoming more visible. For example, the profiles of birthing people in receipt of midwifery care are diversifying in terms of their age, gender, health profile, long-term conditions and social dynamics. Indeed, trans men and nonbinary people are a growing population of childbearing within 'maternity' services. Unlike the term cisgender, used to describe a person who experiences a normative relationship between their gender and sex, *trans* can be used as an umbrella term referring to individuals and groups who do not experience a normative relationship between their gender and sex. Sensitivity to gender diverse folk's experience of navigating systems presently and inadvertently designed to exclude them can allow the profession to redesign and deliver care that is inclusive, and person centred for all. In pursuit of reduced inequalities, we may also decolonise our services where presently white, cisgender, heterosexual and patriarchal norms remain oppressive and exclude diversity. We will explore how we might do this later.

The contemporary midwifery profession is similarly diversifying. Significantly, midwifery is now less mono-gendered, in that men are joining the profession. Yet, how might midwives, who are also men, navigate a profession dominated by women, particularly in a global context where healthcare is typically delivered by women, and yet led by men (World Health Organisation 2019)? The following contemporary insights are offered by John Pendleton, a cisgender man, who is also a midwife and published academic in the field of gender and the midwifery profession.

Surviving and Thriving as a Man Working as a Midwife

Working as a midwife is frequently cited as being a tremendous privilege, and this remains true for men who enter this historically mono-gendered profession. Nevertheless, as relatively recent arrivals we face some unique challenges. In the United Kingdom (UK) we have only been part of the profession for 40 years (Speak and Aitken-Swan 1982) and our presence in the profession was vehemently opposed by all key maternity stakeholders (McKenna 1991). Despite there being no shortage of midwives that necessitated opening up the profession to men, nevertheless legislative changes were driven through bringing the UK into line with EEC directives of 1976 opening the doors for the first pioneers. Globally, men are still banned from midwifery in at least five countries including Japan (Sannomiya et al. 2019).

Into this background of not being wanted or needed, it is perhaps not surprising that men in midwifery are vanishingly rare – currently 0.3% of the UK population (NMC 2019) with similarly low numbers elsewhere. This does present some unique

(continued)

(*continued*)

challenges for us, not least in how to make sense of our experiences. Unlike our counterparts in nursing and allied health professions, we are almost entirely absent from academic literature and empirical enquiry, and the history of men's wider involvement in maternity services is frequently positioned as in conflict with the values and skills of midwives (Pendleton 2019). We also tend to train and work in isolation from other men and there are no professional networks. In fact, from my own research of over 22 hours of interviewing with 15 other men, I learned that there is little appetite to connect with other men. So, the number one strategy for surviving and thriving as a man in midwifery appears to be, keep a low profile! Perhaps because our presence has been so contested and problematic in the past, there is a significant need to assimilate and blend in, to prove we are not there to disrupt or takeover the profession and that we share the same philosophy of care as our female counterparts.

Perhaps the key challenge for us is how the male body is often seen as potentially threatening and needing to be managed, particularly when dealing with touch and intimate care procedures. For men in nursing this can be mitigated by gravitating to areas where more typically masculine traits such as physicality, emergency care and technological prowess are valued. Intimate care, both psychological and physical, for sexually active women and birthing people is a key part of the midwifery remit. From my research there appears to be tacit acceptance that this is acceptable for women who are midwives but must constantly be negotiated in both subtle and overt ways by men. There is no single strategy, but humour may be used to put people at ease along with signalling that you are 'non-threatening' by emphasising that you are either gay or married. Nearly everyone I have talked to cites detailed explanation of procedures in order to overemphasise the clinical nature of intimate touch within a midwifery context. Most employed a combination of these tactics along with others, responding to what the unfolding clinical scenario demanded. There is also a need to exaggerate a capacity for caring to counter essentialist beliefs of gender which hold this trait to be primarily the domain of women. This constant vigilance can be emotionally draining for many men.

In the words of one midwife I have interviewed, as a midwife 'your gender is something that is with you all the time'. In other words, your 'maleness' walks into the room before you and must constantly be negotiated, it is not simply enough to be a competent clinician. The good news is that the men I have talked to, like myself, are passionate about being midwives. Choosing a career that challenges social norms is not something that people accidentally fall into and so acts as a first level filtering mechanism, forcing potential applicants to research the role and consider how they might meet its challenges. Being a student midwife can act as a second filtering process, where men have to pass an additional invisible 'test' to prove their acceptability to both colleagues and service users. Once qualified however, all the men I have spoken to have had fulfilling and rewarding careers. In fact, the other piece of good news is that men working as midwives in purely careerist terms appear to 'thrive'. There are no reliable data about the proportion of men who are midwives working in 'senior' or managerial positions but anecdotally there doesn't appear to be any barriers to our progress. What is not clear is whether this is what most men want, or whether the 'glass escalator' effect (Williams 1992) is, in effect, fast-tracking disproportionately more men into more gender-congruent managerial positions away from the hands-on intimate care which challenges social norms.

Dr John Pendleton; Registered Midwife, & Senior Lecturer at the University of Northampton, UK.

In reading John Pendelton's account above, it is clear that some challenges in relation to gender and the midwifery profession remain. What is less clear is how the presence of men in midwifery may challenge social norms and thus challenge the patriarchy in midwifery work in a context where it is understood as being uniquely 'women's work'. In pursuit of growing the midwifery workforce, it will be important to explore why men in midwifery are/were not wanted. Is it that birth is seen as one of the last things to protect from cisgender men in a world where they have seemingly oppressed cisgender women in everything else? – In which case, reinforcing women's purpose and supporting role being solely in reproduction may only serve to reinforce the patriarchal systems and structures which oppress and confine them.

Gender plays an integral part in perpetuating inequalities, and there is arguably no profession or practice more highly gendered than that of midwifery. This gives midwives unique leverage to thrive in making a significant impact on contemporary inequalities around the world. The archaic gender/sex binary systems (woman/female and men/male) currently in place were first manufactured by European settlers (among earlier others) to position white heteropatriarchy as the pinnacle of civilisation (Lugones 2010; Morgensen 2011). In this system, cisgender heterosexual men have been given systemic authority over cisgender women and all other identities. This system is patriarchal, because within this system, men hold the power, and women are largely excluded from power. This may result in direct harm in reproduction (e.g. obstetric violence and/or reproductive control). Patriarchal notions of sex and gender are also racialised and sexualised at their foundations. For example, think of how women from Asia are stereotyped to be sexually submissive, or how Black men are stereotyped as having overly large genitals. Patriarchal systems harm us all (cisgender men too!), by reinforcing ideas about what we should/shouldn't be and what we should/shouldn't do or have according to our gender. We suggest it is futile to fight inequalities from within such a patriarchal system. It must first be deconstructed.

How?

Challenging gender binaries is deconstructive of these patriarchal systems and is therefore also anticolonial (Morgensen 2012; O'Sullivan 2021). It is not only cisgender women who birth, and it is not useful to centre this gender above any other in childbearing. In fact, centring women may only further serve to ingrain them in a binary system which further perpetuates the oppressive patriarchal structures we see at work every day in perinatal services. Just as grouping cars and motorbikes together as 'vehicles' does not erase the individual nature of either, the use of inclusive language in reproductive services equally does not erase cisgender women or anyone else who births. Thus, in contemporary midwifery practice, where gender in relation to reproduction is highly profiled, we have a unique opportunity to be inclusive of all genders and thus thrive in reducing inequalities for all in future 'people-centred' services.

Unfortunately, recent research suggests that some contemporary perinatal services are not very gender inclusive. Research findings highlight how trans men and nonbinary people who decide to reproduce do so within services designed to exclude them (Pezaro et al. 2023). Essentially, 'maternity care' is structured 'around a heteronormative model of care, as the language of "Mum" and "Dad", "husband", "woman"' is ingrained in everyday practices. Even the word midwife is translated to mean 'with woman' and therefore fails to be inclusive where it is not only cisgender women who give birth. Most midwives contributing to this research wanted to be inclusive of all birthing populations but found that contemporary services and systems presented barriers for inclusivity. Ultimately, cisgender, and heteropatriarchal services, administrative procedures, structural forces and interpersonal treatment combine in the perinatal space. Yet such institutionalised 'support' is designed to reinforce a gendered experience of pregnancy and childbirth that marginalises childbearing trans and nonbinary people who do not conform to cisgender ideals. Overall, contemporary providers' stances inform mundane cisgenderism, passive eugenics, stigma visibility, the minority stress model and the 'doing' and 'undoing' of gender. Moreover, midwives reported transphobia apparent among colleagues. Such aversity to those who challenge the gender binaries only serves to reinforce the patriarchal structures in which cisgender women (and others) are harmed. This gives us an opportunity to reimagine a more utopian future for midwifery, leading the way for equality.

Whilst historically, midwives have many achievements to celebrate, contemporaneously there remain challenges in relation to midwives' professional wellbeing and identity, and growing complexities and dynamics in the health and identities of people who birth. It is crucial that midwives are prepared not just to survive, but to thrive in a digital, diverse, dynamic and exciting future. In learning from our past, we may shape our future. In challenging gender binaries in contemporary and historical midwifery and society, midwives may also be anticolonial and thrive in achieving greater reproductive and gestational justice for all (Chadwick 2022; Morison 2021). In learning to unlock their potential, develop healthy coping strategies and navigate complex working environments, midwives can change the world. The vision for this book is to serve as a resource of both personal and professional enablement, enlightenment and advancement for those who seek it.

WHAT TO EXPECT FROM THIS BOOK

In each chapter of this book, we will be inviting you to engage in activities designed to support you to survive and thrive in midwifery. You may want to repeat the activities, return to them later or simply reflect upon them as you complete them. By the end of this book, we hope that all the activities you have engaged in will form a toolkit from which to draw at various stages in your midwifery career. These activities will be personal to you. As such, they will allow you to explore and reach your own personal midwifery goals, which may indeed change over time. Throughout, we encourage you to spend some real quality time investing in yourself with these activities. When you have completed them all, we would love to hear about how they have enabled you, and other midwives, to thrive.

CHAPTER 2

Unearthing Your Identity as a Midwife

INTRO TO CHAPTER

In this chapter, we will explore your personal identity, values and vision and how these might be used to map your own professional journey through midwifery. We will also explore how you might 'find your community', become self-aware to develop personally and professionally as you construct your own personal vision statement as a baseline for decision-making. Throughout this chapter, we use personal examples alongside examples from midwives around the world to illustrate the ideas presented. You may wish to return to this chapter repeatedly as you continue to reflect throughout this book and beyond.

PERSONAL IDENTITY, VALUES AND VISION

Before reading any further, spend a few moments considering the question, 'Who am I?' Take a piece of paper and write down as many responses as you can (aim for up to 20). Once you are finished, put the piece of paper to one side as we will revisit it later in the chapter.

Who we feel we are and our beliefs about ourselves guide our behaviour. Various aspects of our lives converge to bring an overarching *sense* of self. How we see ourselves evolves over time as life events and experiences add to or challenge our beliefs. During specific moments and activities, certain aspects of our *selves* can become more significant, highlighting the complex and multi-faceted nature of identity.

Surviving and Thriving in Midwifery, First Edition. Sally Pezaro and Karen Maher.
© 2025 John Wiley & Sons Ltd. Published 2025 by John Wiley & Sons Ltd.

Our personal identity is shaped by the distinct roles that we take. The groups to which we belong and others within these groups or roles share certain characteristics with us. These shared characteristics are recognisable by others as belonging to that group and our awareness of them feeds into our sense of self. For example, I (Karen) am a mother, an academic, a psychologist, a partner, a female, white British, heterosexual, open-water swimmer and dance music enthusiast. I (Sally) am a parent, a midwife, an academic, a partner, an online gamer and a history fan. Amongst other roles and identities, each of those characteristics/roles/identities shape the beliefs we hold about ourselves through the shared understanding of each of those roles/groups. There are certain normative behaviours expected within each of these roles (e.g. caring and nurturing as a mother, hard-working and task oriented as an academic) and sometimes they may be in conflict which has consequences for how we feel. Particular roles may hold greater importance for us over others and therefore have a greater influence on our sense of self and identity. Those roles and groups which hold greater importance for our identity have greater potential to impact our well-being when challenged or taken away, for example if we hold our job role as playing a significant role in who we are as a person then retirement can be particularly difficult to navigate in terms of our identity. However, these shared characteristics may not always be fixed and stable, as they may be shaped by our expectations based on prior experience but also on other people's expectations of what it means to be a member of that group. So, my (Karen's) identity and expectations of what it means to be a mother will be shaped by my experience of being mothered, my understanding of watching others being mothers and the expectations of others on my own mothering. For you (and Sally), your identity, and expectations of what it means to be a midwife will be shaped by your prior experiences with midwives (be that through being supported in your own birth experience, having midwives in your social network or through portrayals of midwifery in media), and the expectations of you as a midwife by others.

The roles and groups to which we associate shape our understanding of ourselves. One way this happens is through others reflecting back our identities. The Looking Glass Self is a concept first presented in the early twentieth century to suggest social interaction is a form of 'mirror' reflecting judgements and perceptions from others back to us which influence our thoughts about ourselves and, consequently, our behaviour (Cooley 1902). The messages we get from others about the roles and attributes we hold important can have both positive and negative effects. An example of this could be when giving a presentation. You may start feeling confident and positive cues from the audience such as nodding and smiling can increase your confidence and leave you feeling good about your performance. However, if the audience gives you negative cues such as yawning or looking at their phone or watches, this may impact your confidence and how good you feel you are at giving presentations. Of particular importance to midwifery is how others view the profession (from allied professions, those within your care and the wider public and media) as all this forms part of your personal 'looking glass'. Whilst it is not possible to control the thoughts and behaviours of others, having an awareness of how it influences your own personal narrative about yourself can be a powerful first step in reducing the impact of negative judgements and perceptions.

As well as the roles and groups of which we are part, our personality is often thought of as part of what makes us unique individuals. Our personality can be understood as those thoughts, feelings and behaviours that make us who we are. In mainstream psychology, there are schools of thought which attempt to prescribe specific traits and attributes to individuals with the suggestion that such traits are stable, fixed and measurable. This has found its way into everyday understandings of personality seen by people labelling themselves as introvert/extrovert, empathic, neurotic, etc. However, taking this fixed approach fails to capture the nuance in our personalities over time and in certain situations. For example, I (Karen) display extroverted behaviour in small groups but introverted behaviour when in large groups. Seeing personality as more dynamic than simply pigeonholing people into neat little boxes allows for a richer expression of ourselves and the acknowledgement of how our experiences shape our understanding of who we are. Transitions in life such as starting to train to become a midwife, taking on a leadership position, becoming a parent, significant bereavements, amongst others, influence those thoughts, feelings and behaviours which make up our personality. Through awareness of our thoughts, feelings and behaviours and their relationship with our life experiences we can gain a sense of an authentic or 'true' self (discussed later in this chapter). Part of this authentic self can relate to specific traits or attributes that you associate with yourself (such as empathy, assertiveness, confidence, shyness, etc.); part can relate to those skills and abilities we believe we have (such as communication skills, organisation skills, specific clinical skills or educational skills) and part can relate to more transient aspects of ourselves such as appearance, job role and personal interests. The degree to which each part influences how we see ourselves will depend on the situation and what we hold as important at any given moment in time.

One core aspect of our personality that guides our behaviour are our values. Values are learned beliefs about how we should act and how the world should be. They are a socially constructed part of our personality shaped by our environment. Values guide our behaviour through having a motivational element, they determine what goals and outcomes to strive for. We hold several values which have relative importance to each other within a value system which means there can sometimes be conflict. For example, you may place high value on achievement (through gaining promotion at work, or winning awards/accolades, completing further study for self-improvement) but also value benevolence and helping others. The behaviours required for the former can often conflict with the latter (e.g. gaining a promotion or winning an award may put you in competition with a friend/colleague, completing further study may mean reducing hours at work leaving your team under resourced). Therefore, having knowledge of our values and the relative importance of each against the others we can have a clearer idea of what goals to set for ourselves (see Chapter 9) and feel more comfortable with the decisions we make. When there is discomfort or unease about a decision or our behaviour it may arise from a conflict with our values. However, when practising within our values we can make tough choices, have challenging conversations and do courageous things, but the first step is to know what our own values are. As such, there will be an opportunity to gain insight into your own personal values when discussing self-awareness later in this chapter.

The value system we hold helps us develop our personal 'brand' or our 'vision'. Our vision is what we stand for in all aspects of our lives. It is linked to our personal identity and who we are, but it is more than that. It is the guiding light for all that we do, not just in midwifery, but with our families, friends, when we visit the shops and in our leisure activities. In the same way that an organisation or business has a vision (your place of work should have one and it would be worth searching this out as it will give you an idea of how your role adds to the organisation's vision and give you a sense of how well your values align with your organisation's), and that vision guides the strategic choices of the organisation and where to invest its time and resources, your personal vision should do the same. The more time, energy and resources we invest in our personal vision, the more positive our well-being and satisfaction with life will be. A vision statement is often broad and not set around specific goals or objectives but serves as a general guide. My own (Karen's) vision is to support and empower others to be happy, healthy and content versions of themselves. This has guided my educational choices, the jobs I have applied for and taken, the research I do, how I parent my children, my relationships with my friends and family and the leisure activities I take part in. After identifying your values take some time to consider how these relate and shape your own personal vision and your professional journey.

NAVIGATING YOUR PROFESSIONAL JOURNEY

The perception often can be that being a midwife is all about catching babies. It is true indeed that every birth is touched by a midwife, yet this touch is not always a physical one. Sometimes our influence is carried via a variety of non-clinical roles, which in turn enable our profession and influence to grow and flourish in a myriad of ways. When the World Health Organisation (WHO) declared 2020 as the international year of the midwife and nurse I (Sally) detailed how midwives might maximise their opportunities to diversify (Pezaro 2019). In truth, there is no limit to our role in society. Midwives can and should influence all aspects of life. We are awesome.

Some more typical non-clinical roles a midwife may explore are ones in commissioning, consultancy, education, management, policy, quality assurance, regulation and/or research. Yet there are also calls for investment in midwifery leadership and governance positions elsewhere, anywhere where decisions affecting sexual, reproductive, maternal, neonatal and adolescent health (SRMNAH) are being made (Nove et al. 2021). Of course, nobody needs to decide from the beginning of their career where they might end up. Yet it is important to think about what legacy you want to leave, what excites and motivates you and where you might best thrive.

As a start, ask yourself, 'where might I be in 5 years' time?' In Chapter 9 we will help you set goals to get there.

Every midwifery journey is different. Yet whichever path you choose on your professional journey, it can be exceptionally challenging to survive and thrive in the midwifery profession at times. This is partly why we saw a need for this book. Such challenges are often beyond our control, and yet we still need to navigate our way through them or seek different pathways to survival. When we start out as student midwives, we have dreams and ideals of what practising as a midwife might be like.

Yet often our expectations are not matched with reality, or we find it exceptionally challenging to get where we need and want to be. Moreover, the reality is often that our work environments are not conducive to us surviving and thriving. So how might we navigate this in our own professional journey?

With the help of the 'Nursing Now Challenge' (who engage a global network of midwives too!), we reached out to midwives and nurse-midwives across the world and asked them to contribute some of their own professional stories and episodes of where they themselves have survived and thrived. Many of these reflect the diversity and challenges in our careers. We hope you will return to the excerpts below when in need of insight, inspiration and perspective.

> *Working in Nigeria as a midwife was a challenging one for me as most often, we face women who are not well educated, so have no or little knowledge about health, pregnancy, birth and childcare. This required additional effort to educate and guide them all through pregnancy, birth and follow up....*

> *Coming to United Arab Emirates was different case, as it is a medicalized environment, where the physicians are in the lead. This often makes the midwifery job dependent on their orders. Coming to the pandemic, it is quite challenging to stay in an isolation room with a covid-19 positive mother throughout labour with a full PPE. Often these women are emotional... due to their diagnosis [of Covid-19], and so need a lot of emotional support. It has been amazing to see how we have thrived amidst all the challenges to provide care. I now look forward to an independent midwifery practice in the middle east, United Arab Emirates to be precise.*

> – Midwife, United Arab Emirates (From Nigeria)

> *I have been in the NHS since 2007, a midwife since 2016. I left my previous trust because of the bullying culture and felt very unsafe in my work. I have been in my new trust since June 2021 and have never felt so supported and cared for. I feel like the new team I am working with care for me and my well-being, I feel like a valued member of the team, and this has supported me to thrive and not just survive as a midwife.*

> – Practice Educator and Retention Lead Midwife,
> United Kingdom

> *Sharing different opinion and discussions in a same platform with a different Midwives in different countries can help midwives to thrive*

> – Midwife, Somalia

> *I am passionate about safe staff and patient care because they are intrinsically linked. In 2013 I documented unsafe staffing internally and was called a 'vindictive liar' by the Risk Manager, who was also a supervisor of midwives. I chose to submit further Datix [critical incident report] on unsafe staffing and these were escalated within trust. Eventually I was labelled a legitimate internal*

whistle-blower, and the trust apologized. Now I have national PhD funding researching the staff experience of escalation of care in maternity services. Keep speaking your truth and know your boundaries, because they are for you, and you are worth protecting.

– PhD Fellow/Midwifery Lecturer, United Kingdom

In a country like India, we 'Midwives' have the most difficulty to survive as the medical professionals are dominating and the public is more inclined toward the obstetricians. The reasons may be varied, based on the evolutions that happened and doctors wanting to survive, so they don't encourage and support midwives to evolve independently. I am hopeful that efforts are been taken to 'Bring the Midwives back' in India.... If everyone puts their complete efforts to success, then we can change the scenario by influencing self (Midwives), medical fraternity [sic], public, policy level.

– Assistant Professor of Midwifery, India

In order to survive and thrive in Midwifery over the past 18 years, I have had to adapt and embrace many challenges. Despite long working hours; a lack of resources, a lack of direction at times; pay freezes, staff shortages and a tumbling morale, I have never lost sight of WHY I became a midwife in the first place. The closeness, empowerment and respect that I felt towards the powerhouse of a midwife that guided me through the birth of my first child, motivated and inspired me to become a midwife. From that moment my future was set, and I will never regret my decision to become a midwife. It felt like a calling, it still does. At this point in my career, I could step out of clinical midwifery and into management, teaching or a specialism, but I don't want to. I want to be with women and people, I want to empower, guide, motivate and celebrate. I am not saying that it's easy, it not. What I'm saying is that it's worth it.

– Labour ward Midwife/Co-ordinator, United Kingdom

Carry your own chair to the high table. Always learning, never ending ...

– Midwife and Founding Director, Uganda

I have survived and thrived in midwifery by developing a mindset from the phrase' begin with the end in mind'. I believe most of the challenges faced are unique to every setting and country depending on what you are employed to do. Therefore, my focus has always been the legacy I will leave even if what I want to achieve will not come to fruition as planned but I will always be in the history. Developing a thick skin and not being easily discouraged when things are not going as planned. Instead looking for an alternative option or looking at innovative ways to accomplish your aim even if you must meet in the middle with people initially is also another way I've thrived and survived in midwifery.

– Director of nursing and midwifery, Qatar

I survived as a newly qualified midwife by having a strong, supportive team with a shared vision. Head, heart and hands – Innovation and curiosity, compassion and care, action, and joint working.

– Midwife, United Kingdom

I started studying midwifery at certificate level. Immediately I was retained by the training school administrators to assist with teaching midwifery clinicals in the skills Laboratory and clinical supervision in the placement for certificate level students. Due to shortage of staff in the institution, I sometimes found myself extending my arm of service to diploma midwifery students. It was at this time that I realized a need to upgrade to a higher academic level to suit the position of service. After 4 years of service, I studied a diploma in midwifery. I thought the diploma was good enough to suit the quality-of-service delivery in the place not until when I got the opportunity to participate in LUGINA AFRICA MIDWIFERY RESEARCH NETWORK (LAMRAN) research meetings!

The inspiration to study and advance in midwifery: *The meetings gave me a chance to interact with both national and international midwives who had studied and advanced in midwifery and research. People had bachelor's degrees, masters, fellowships, PhDs! Wow, Wow! I was so amazed! The research language sounded so new! It was from these interactions with the learned midwives that I was inspired to study more and specialize in midwifery and research.*

The academic advancement journey: *The journey to attainment of a bachelor's degree in midwifery was not easy given the fact that the program had not yet started in Uganda. I had no support for an international program. There was a bachelor's in nursing which was only being offered to only nurse with diplomas but strictly not midwives. I felt blocked by the policy but counselled myself and studied a diploma in Nursing to qualify for bachelor's admission entry criteria.*

Current academic progress: *Currently I have bachelor's degree in Nursing, I have just completed a master's degree in Midwifery and women's Health at Makerere University, School of Health Sciences, Uganda. I am pursuing a nine-month post graduate diploma in medical education (PGD Med) at Makerere University, as I wait for my master's degree graduation. I hope to start a PhD in midwifery and women's Health by academic year 2023.*

Research progress: *My master's degree research thesis focused on 'Assessing the competence of midwives in assisting frank breech vaginal births' in lower-level health centers. I have submitted this thesis to Makerere University, as a requirement for the award of a master's degree in midwifery and women's health. At the same time, I am working on a manuscript for publication of the study findings.*

Achievement: I have taught midwifery to many students where many have qualified with certificates and diplomas and are employed in various hospitals delivering quality evidence-based midwifery services. I have just been employed as a midwifery assistant lecturer at Uganda Christian University. This has given me a chance to teach midwifery at bachelor's degree level! I aim to teach at more advanced levels (Masters and PhD) with the attainment of more specialized education and training. I have acquired more research knowledge and yearn to participate in midwifery research both nationally and internationally. I hope to supervise midwifery students' research projects for academic award.

– Midwifery educator, Uganda

Thank you to every contributor for their powerful words here. It is important to keep sharing such stories to both capture and remember our experiences, but also to know that none of us are alone in our diversity of experience.

When you do have direction in your professional journey, it will be important to seize relevant opportunities for training wherever possible, particularly in leadership. If you see a position you wish to aspire to, check out the job description and what the pre-requisites are for the job you want. Then set goals and source ways in which to achieve them (more on this later). In this pursuit, networking is always helpful. Talk to and gravitate towards those you can learn from.

Also be aware that your own professional journey could be a one for others to follow. Share your own successes along the way. Leave footprints large enough for someone else to easily step into those you leave behind. We hope we are doing that here in this book.

FINDING YOUR CHOSEN COMMUNITY

To thrive, it is important to get yourself into and remain in psychologically safe spaces (see Chapter 5 for a more in-depth discussion on psychological safety). The people around you can affect you both positively and/or negatively, and it is important to remain aware of this as you unearth your own professional identity and thrive in midwifery.

Now, when we say 'chosen community' we do not mean some exclusive club or 'clique' where only people considered part of a certain elite are welcomed. Nevertheless, through the lens of social identity theory, members of a professional group can observe power and authority gradients whereby one group is seen to have power over another, and more often see the attributes of their own professional group as positive and those of other professional groups as less desirable (Weller 2012). This can, in turn, lead to the development of derogatory and/or incorrect stereotypes. Such tribalism and power gradients can also have a negative impact upon one's feeling of value and being able to escalate concerns safely, leaving poor decisions to go unchecked.

Though our professional identity as midwives may be strong, we also need to identify as part of the wider health care team. This can happen more effectively when work is organised around the multidisciplinary team looking after people who birth in our services rather than being organised around a specific professional team based upon a single professional group. In this sense, we all need to shift our thinking towards working in this way, so that our multidisciplinary community may thrive.

On an individual level, you may need to find a more bespoke community in which to thrive. In this, it is important to think about who may be most aligned to your values and vision for the future. For example, if you are continually being told 'no' by a midwifery colleague in response to your ideas, without good reason, that person may not be best suited to sit within your community. Yet someone who respectfully challenges you, poses alternatives and/or invites you to think more deeply or ambitiously about things may enrich you both personally and professionally by sitting in your community. People who just agree with you all the time are not always the best fit! It is also important to go where you are celebrated.

In midwifery, social media has always been a wonderful place to 'find your community'. You can find us on X, TikTok or LinkedIn, say 'Hi' and we can introduce you to some top midwifery folk (@SallyPezaro & @karenmaher76).

Whilst it is always encouraging to have mentors and coaches around to share their expertise with you, what every midwife really needs is a champion. Someone to truly cheer them on and help them realise their full potential. Generally, being around people who make you feel confident and emboldened to fulfil your destiny are those worthy of being in your community. Choose carefully and be kind to those who need to leave your chosen community at any time, for they have no doubt enriched you through lessons learnt too.

Networks are also key in accomplishing tasks and achieving both personal and organisational goals (Ibarra and Hunter 2007). Three related but distinct types of connections are particularly instrumental in this task:

- **Strategic network:** These comprise diverse connections with disparate affiliations and objectives which can be leveraged to promote support for ideas, and secure the resources needed for realising goals.
- **Personal network:** These are like-minded connections outside of work who can provide you with insight and new perspectives to help you in advancing your career. They may also provide opportunities for mentorship and/or coaching.
- **Operational network:** These connections help you get the job done. They are inwardly focused, and task oriented.

Finally in relation to your chosen community, remember that you can also influence your community and others by the way in which you conduct yourself. You need to ensure that your community is a welcoming role model for others to aspire to, rather than an exclusive community wielding its power to bring others down. In this pursuit, self-awareness is key.

SELF-AWARENESS AND PERSONAL DEVELOPMENT

At the start of this chapter, we provided an overview of personal identity and how this relates to our values and personal vision. Self-awareness is the processes of gaining insight into what that means for us. What are the distinct roles and groups that shape my identity? What attributes and traits do I have and how do they influence my behaviour? What values do I hold important and how do these influence the goals I make for myself? What is the guiding light leading me towards my decisions (my personal vision)? It has been a topic of contemplation, discussion and guidance for centuries from Greek philosophy, religious scholars and spiritual guides to psychologists, academics and contemporary self-help gurus. As Carl Jung, one of the most influential psychologists and psychoanalysts of our time, so succinctly puts it;

Your visions will become clear only when you can look into your own heart...
Who looks outside, dreams; who looks inside, awakes.

(Jung 1973, Letters Vol. 1, p. 33)

Self-awareness can be defined as *'the will and the skill to understand yourself and how others see you'* (Eurich 2017, p. 24). This definition implies there needs to be an intention and desire to be self-aware as well as having the necessary abilities and resources to make it happen. There is also the consideration of the internal world (our thoughts, feelings, motivators, temperament, etc.) and the external world (how others perceive us). However, a balance is needed between the internal and the external. Too little self-knowledge can lead to living in a way that is unfulfilling and misaligned to your core values but too much introspection can become self-absorption without understanding the impact you have on those around you. Too little understanding of how others see you can mean it is difficult to understand and take on feedback but too much can bring rumination and placing an unhelpful emphasis on what others think.

Self-awareness is a process of internal evaluation and must come before any personal development; how do you know what you need to work on without insight into your strengths, weaknesses, challenges and what you hold as important? Self-awareness involves asking lots of questions and being curious about how we navigate our environment. It allows for an evaluation of our current self, identification of our ideal self and an understanding of the gap between the two. The narrower the gap between our current self and our ideal self the better our self-esteem and the greater the feeling of being *authentic*. Self-awareness also allows for an evaluation of how we see ourselves versus how others see us, and again, the more aligned they are the greater the feeling of authenticity. Increased self-awareness has been linked to increased confidence, stronger relationships, more ethical and moral behaviours, greater job satisfaction and increased chance of promotion (Bass and Yammarino 1991; Fletcher and Bailey 2003; Silvia and O'Brien 2004; Wexley et al. 1980). When asked, most people would state that they are self-aware and know themselves, however, when tested empirically, only 10–15% of people met the criteria for self-awareness (Eurich 2017).

We asked you at the start to write down up to 20 responses to the question 'Who am I?'. Hopefully, you still have the piece of paper to hand so spend a few moments looking over your answers. Reflect on which ones are related to roles/group membership, which are traits and attributes, which are feelings/emotions/thoughts. Do any of the responses hold greater importance over the others? If so, what makes them more important?

However, self-awareness is only part of the process towards personal growth. Personal development centres on those activities we engage in that move us closer to our authentic self. Using action planning and goal setting (see Chapter 9) we can move towards a life, both in midwifery and outside, that is fulfilling and aligned to our authentic self.

TOOLS FOR SELF-AWARENESS AND PERSONAL DEVELOPMENT

Whilst there are many tools, questionnaires and activities, we can use to enhance self-awareness, the one thing that underpins all of them is our own curiosity to learn about ourselves. As part of midwifery training and ongoing professional development there is a need to engage in reflective practice. The purpose of reflective practice is to think critically and evaluatively about your professional experience to adapt, learn and grow as a midwife (and person). This same process can be applied when developing self-awareness, but you are expanding the reflection outwards beyond the work environment to all aspects of your life. With reflective practice the outcome of the process is to identify an action plan for professional development, and so it stands that the outcome of self-awareness practices should be an action plan to move you closer towards your authentic self. The reflective goal setting framework in Chapter 9 provides one way to structure this process.

There are many tools you can use to help with developing personal insight and the following is not an exhaustive list of tools, but good starting points based on evidence about what works.

Values in Action Strengths tool (VIA): This is a self-assessment tool to explore your character strengths which allows us to see the positive aspects of our personality. When living and working within our strengths we can protect our well-being and have a greater sense of purpose and fulfilment. www.viacharacter.org

Journaling and reflective/expressive writing: Journaling has been often cited as a way to process and make sense of our thoughts and experiences; however, this comes with a caveat. Simply writing about what has happened over the course of a day or focussing on the positive (e.g. gratitude diaries) has benefits for our well-being but comes at the expense of self-awareness. If we write about our negative experiences, whilst difficult and potentially emotionally painful at the time, it can lead to greater insight into what happened, what sense we can make of it and what actions we can take in the future which could lead to more productive outcomes (Pennebaker 1997). It should be a way to process our thoughts and feelings rather than a pressure release valve for venting emotions or a rose-tinted view of the day. Benefits of journaling in this way can be achieved by writing a couple of days per week and you are aiming for quality rather than quantity; writing every day runs the risk of rumination and self-absorption, so take time to reflect on what you have written before writing the next entry.

Meditation/mindfulness: Mindfulness is one of those words in modern vocabulary that can receive a mixed reaction through perceived associations. Simply put mindfulness is the opposite of mindlessness and the modern world is geared up for lots of mindlessness. We often run on autopilot and make cognitive shortcuts in the process, meaning we miss novelty, learning opportunities, creativity, alternative solutions to problems and the rich tapestry of life around us. By way of a definition, mindfulness is *paying attention, on purpose, without judgement* and is the process of noticing our thoughts, feelings, behaviours without labelling them or reacting to them. We can do this by purposefully attending to where we are and what we are doing at any given moment and noticing the thoughts and feelings that arise (imagine it being like watching your thoughts on a TV screen). Meditation is one way we can strengthen that mindfulness muscle. Engaging in meditative practice is the mental equivalent of going to the gym making it easier to be mindful in our everyday life, but even without meditation, the more we purposefully attend to our lives the more mindful we become. So, what does that have to do with self-awareness? By attending to our thoughts, feelings, and behaviours in the moment and viewing them as a neutral observer we can make sense of our place in the world; so we gain insight without the navel-gazing and rumination.

Feedback: Gaining as much feedback as we can from others gives us a broader picture of the way others perceive us. However, getting feedback is often a tricky process as those closest to us may not always give us the full picture though for fear of hurting our feelings and, at work, people may not feel adequately skilled to give useful feedback, even if they are in leadership roles. In addition, there is a need for you, as the receiver of feedback, to remain open to all potential feedback offered, however unpalatable it may feel at the time. And so structured feedback processes such as performance appraisals can sometimes provide a safe place for gaining feedback but usually this happens with your line manager so can feel quite one-dimensional. A more advanced version of the performance appraisal is 360 feedback whereby feedback is offered from all levels of people you interact with at work both horizontally and vertically. Therefore, you can gain feedback not only from your line manager, but the colleagues in your team both midwives and those from allied professions and anyone you have responsibility for, such as student midwives. If your organisation offers this process, you may find it a useful reference point, however, feedback from different directions may not always be consistent and may even contradict each other. We are also keen to acknowledge that these formal forms of feedback and appraisal may not always be supportive, useful or positive experiences. If this is the case, then your community can be a reliable source of feedback, particularly those within your community with whom you have mutual trust and where you wish the best for each other. When gaining feedback from your community it is important to be specific about what you want feedback on (specific characteristics, performance or behaviours) and how you would like the feedback interaction to happen (over dinner/coffee, on the telephone, while out for a walk, via email/text). Other ways of gaining feedback on which to reflect would be old school reports or training placement reports. These can give insight on potential areas for development that might still be hanging around as well as a point of reflection as to how far you have grown as a person and professional midwife.

The Values Bullseye

Earlier we discussed the importance of values for shaping your personal vision and understanding your personality. The Values Bullseye (Lundgren et al. 2012) is a tool designed to become aware of your values and how they are reflected within your life (see Figure 2.1). In the appendix is an extensive list of potential values. It is not an exhaustive list, but it gives a flavour of the sorts of things considered values and there is space for you to add extras that you feel fit more appropriately for you. Using that list as a starting point write down your values for each of the four sections of the bullseye. What matters to you in each of those domains? What sort of person do you want to be? What personal qualities do you want to develop?

Work and Education (refers to your workplace and career, education, knowledge, skill development including volunteering or other unpaid work)

Leisure (refers to how you play, relax, stimulate or enjoy yourself including hobbies and other activities)

Relationships (refers to intimacy, closeness, friendship and bonding including relationships with partner, spouse, children, parents and other relatives, friends, colleagues and other social contacts)

Personal Growth and health (refers to your ongoing development as a human being including religion/spirituality, physical health and well-being, life skills, self-care)

Reflecting on your answers in each of the sections above consider where you stand today in living in tune with those values. On the dart board below make an X to represent where you are in each domain; an X in the centre of the board means you are living fully in line with those values, whereas an X on the outer circle means you have lost touch with the values in that area. In total, you should have four X on the board.

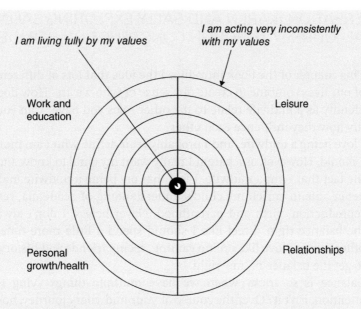

FIGURE 2.1   Values Bullseye. *Source*: adapted from Lundgren et al. (2012).

Once you have identified where you currently are in relation to your values, consider what barriers and obstacles are preventing you from living life fully by your values. What gets in the way of living the kind of life that is consistent with your values? Write any obstacles below and rate them on a 1–7 scale (1 = does not prevent me at all, 7 = prevents me completely).

The last step is to create an action plan that moves you towards living fully within your values for each domain in your life and can be used in conjunction with Reflective Goal Setting presented in Chapter 9. Consider what actions you can take in your daily life to overcome the barriers and obstacles you identified. Identify one value-based action that you can do this week in each of the four domains. Using small incremental actions can keep your plan manageable and prevent feeling overwhelmed if there is a long way to travel. Write your actions in each domain below.

Work and Education:

Leisure and Recreation:

Personal Growth and Health:

Relationships:

IN CONVERSATION (KAREN AND SALLY EXPLORING SALLY'S PERSONAL JOURNEY THROUGH CONSTRUCTING HER IDENTITY)

KM   This chapter of the book introduced the idea that lots of different areas of our lives combine to create our sense of who we are. How does your identity as a midwife relate to the other roles you have? Can you identify how they influence each other?

SP   I love being a midwife, and I probably let it define who I am more than I should. However, as a parent I really want my child to know and value the fact that I am a midwife. I feel that my being a midwife makes me better able to enrich my child's understanding of academia, research, reproduction, birth and parenthood. Nevertheless, I don't always get the balance right. I feel like I should spend a little more time doing other things I love like online gaming, seeing friends and history walks to get the balance of 'me' right.

KM   Balance is so tricky when we have multiple things vying for our attention, isn't it? Over the course of your midwifery journey, how have other people's perceptions of midwifery shaped your identity?

SP   I have heard many falsehoods about midwifery in my time. My Grandpa was a nurse and would say to me, 'when are you going to move on from midwifery to become a full nurse?' as if I wasn't already in my own specialist area.

Even now, other friends and family say to me… 'Do you think you will ever go back to midwifery?' Yet I actually feel more involved with midwifery now that I am practising in research and academia than I ever did when I was practising clinically. That's a personal thing, I think.

In terms of finding **my** community, I have always thrived where I am celebrated and where I feel respected and valued. So, my community tends to include people who lift others as they climb and stay away from negativity and incivility. The midwifery profession needs us all to thrive, and I know that I don't thrive where I don't feel psychologically safe. So, I stay away from people who threaten my psychological safety. I can't let people shame or victimise me, and so my community is generally solution focussed and maintains a high level of psychological safety.

KM   It is interesting that you highlight psychological safety as it is really important in teams. It gives space for creativity, to be able to try out new ideas without fear of negative consequences. We will talk about this in more detail later so thinking back to your identity as a midwife, how has the way you have chosen to work helped to shape your professional identity?

SP   Whilst I have a strong professional identity, I very much enjoy working collaboratively with non-midwives. I think you must be quite confident to do this, but it certainly enriches your thinking, especially when you bring different perspectives together in solving a problem.

KM   I completely agree. A lot of knowledge and ways of doing things we take for granted and these can be challenged when working with people from other disciplines. This can give deeper insight not only on the problem you are working with, but also on yourself, who you are and the way you work. With that in mind, in what ways have your values shaped the decisions and choices you have made in your career, such as working with non-midwives or taking an academic focus?

SP   I have always marvelled at birth and the process of childbearing. Yet clinical midwifery practice did not align with what I needed to thrive. This was largely because I didn't experience the clinical workplace as being psychologically safe. In fact, I found it decidedly psychologically unsafe. Yet as my values strongly align with being an evidence-based practitioner, I had a powerful desire to generate and use the evidence needed for enhancing midwifery and move into research and academia. In addition, being an educationalist aligns with my vision to enable others to thrive. Consequently, I am thriving as a midwife academic in research and education far more now than I ever did in clinical midwifery practice earlier on in my career. I also have a far more enriching community around me now than I have ever had before. The best is yet to come.

Activity – Constructing Your Personal Vision Statement

The different self-awareness tools presented towards the end of the chapter provide access to various aspects of yourself. Take some time to go through as many of these activities as you wish to gain insight into what motivates you and guides your decision-making. With this insight, use the space below to write your personal vision statement. Keep in mind it should be broad and relate to all aspects of your life, not just your professional life. When tough decisions need to be made reflect on your personal vision and identify the ways in which all potential options move you towards your vision (or not).

_____

_____

_____

_____

_____

_____

CHAPTER 3

Surviving and Thriving the Day to Day

INTRO TO CHAPTER

Surviving and thriving the day to day in midwifery practice can be extremely challenging. There is a call for more comprehensive and systematic interventions to promote staff well-being within healthcare, rather than focusing on individual employees. If you have a management or influential role within your own organisation, we recommend exploring the implementation of organisational level interventions as these are typically shown to have better effectiveness than individual level ones. In the resources section, we have included some key readings which can provide guidance on the design of organisational level interventions. However, our aim for this book is to provide a toolkit to navigate your own surviving and thriving. Therefore, this chapter explores some of the day-to-day challenges midwives face on an individual level.

In response to the COVID-19 pandemic, the 'Humans Not Heroes' project emerged as a collaboration between academics at Coventry University and China Plate Theatre in the UK. This project has thus far seen five cohorts of healthcare workers each co-creating an audio artwork based on their experiences of working throughout the ongoing pandemic. Participants have come from a variety of roles and experiences.

In December 2021, the Humans Not Heroes team premiered the first in the latest series of artwork as part of 'Coventry Creates' an initiative established as Coventry became UK City of Culture 2021. This work was funded by The Rayne Foundation and Winston Churchill Memorial Trust. To gain a sense of what it is like to work clinically

Surviving and Thriving in Midwifery, First Edition. Sally Pezaro and Karen Maher.
© 2025 John Wiley & Sons Ltd. Published 2025 by John Wiley & Sons Ltd.

and manage the demands of the day to day in healthcare services, you can access and listen to all the audio artworks via the QR codes below.

With some of those day-to-day challenges in mind from the project, in this chapter, we will explore how you might manage the demands of working in midwifery and protect your resources. We will also explore how you can maintain compassion and optimise shift work. Lastly, we will share some insights as to how you might thrive and survive in 'midwifing outside the system'.

MANAGING DEMANDS AND PROTECTING RESOURCES

Well-being, as defined by the World Health Organisation, is where 'every individual realizes his or her own potential, can cope with the normal stresses of life, can work productively and fruitfully, and is able to make a contribution to her or his community' (World Health Organisation 2022a). From a work perspective, well-being can be the balance between our work demands (the tasks we must do, the way we do them and how long we have to complete them) and the resources we have available to complete them. When there is an imbalance, we can experience the negative emotions associated with stress which, if prolonged, can lead to burnout.

Stress and burnout are hot topics within midwifery. Prior to the COVID-19 pandemic concerns had been raised regarding the well-being of the midwifery work-force (Royal College of Midwives 2017) with a vicious cycle of high workloads leading to midwives leaving the profession which in turn leads to higher workloads for those who remain. In 2016, nearly half of those surveyed by the RCM reported feeling stressed either every day or most days. Since then, pressures have increased due to the COVID-19 pandemic (Kinman et al. 2020) with the effects likely to be felt for years to come due to the time taken to train new recruits to plug the existing gaps. Whilst tackling those structural issues within midwifery is key to long-term protection of the midwifery workforce against burnout and stress (Royal College of Midwives 2017), there are practical steps each individual midwife can take to effectively manage and cope in their working life in the meantime.

Stress is one of those concepts that is used so much in common language that often we think we are sharing a collective understanding and definition, but sometimes that is not the case. Within the academic literature there is often disagreement but, for the purposes of this book, the Health and Safety Executive (HSE) has a good working definition that helps to understand the mechanisms of stress in the workplace.

> *Stress is the adverse reaction people have to excessive pressures and other types of demands placed upon them... Workers feel stress when they can't cope with pressures and other issues. (Health and Safety Executive 2019)*

There is a difference between stress and pressure, with pressure being a motivational force driving us towards high performance. Stress occurs when this pressure becomes excessive, and we are no longer able to cope. The HSE definition highlights the role that work plays in our experience of stress with certain work conditions strongly linked to work-related stress.

- Demands: including workload, shift patterns and physical work environment.
- Control: how much say you have over the way you do your job.
- Support: the encouragement and resources provided by your line manager, colleagues and the wider organisation including training, feedback and mentoring.
- Relationships: are there positive relationships at work? Are issues of conflict and unacceptable behaviour dealt with quickly and effectively?
- Role: how well you understand what is expected of you within your role and if there is any conflict between different aspects of your role.
- Change: the effectiveness of the management and communication of organisational change within the organisation.

Some of those work conditions are structural and any change in issues such as how conflict is dealt with, or the communication and management of change maybe outside the influence of many front-line clinically based midwives. But some aspects can be influenced, particularly around the demands and resources we encounter within our work lives, and in some respects our non-work lives.

Demands at work are those things which require either psychological or physical effort, therefore depleting energy. Within midwifery, at the present time the demands at work are high with large caseloads of people within the care of individual midwives, who may be dealing with multiple births simultaneously, impacting on the type of care they wish to give or is seen as best practice. These competing demands can lead to a conflict between the role you have to do versus the role you want to do, e.g. building trusting relationships with those in your care to have as optimal birthing experience as possible.

When it comes to viewing the work demands within midwifery, it is important to distinguish between hindrance demands and challenge demands. Hindrance demands are those that get in the way of effective performance or can prevent learning and development, for example having to provide care for several people in the latter stages of labour at the same time or not having senior staff available to support you during an obstetric emergency. On the other hand, challenge demands are those that provide opportunities for success and professional growth, for example providing support during a complex birth or using a new technique with experienced support on hand. Whilst both types of demands require energy and so can be depleting in excess, hindrance demands if left unchecked have a greater negative effect on our well-being than challenge demands.

When using stress as the measure of well-being, there is a focus on the absence of ill-health which can mean the more positive aspects of personal growth, happiness and flourishing are overlooked. If we have the resources both at work and within ourselves to buffer the demands of work, we can activate a motivational process leading to increased levels of engagement and thriving at work. Resources are those things which are either useful for achieving work goals, reduce work demands or stimulate personal growth. Examples of resources are having social support within your team at work and/or in your personal life (see Chapter 2 – finding your community), having the right equipment to do your job or career development opportunities. We also have internal personal resources that can help with how job demands impact on us, such as having an optimistic disposition, pro-active coping and certain personality traits such as high emotional stability, amongst others.

The following are actions that can either help manage demands or provide/protect resources at work. Managing demands:

- Job crafting – This relates to minor changes in your work that can influence the degree to which demands may impact upon you and can be seen as a way of increasing challenge demands for personal growth or increasing resources to protect against hindrance demands (Tims et al. 2012). Wrzesniewski and Dutton (2001) categorise job crafting into three areas (i) task crafting (changing aspects of the task itself to make it less demanding, e.g. setting up a new community clinic to reduce the number of individual home visits required), (ii) relational crafting (changing the relationships we have at work to make work less demanding, e.g. working the same shifts as a work friend or mentor), (iii) cognitive crafting (changing the way we think about a task to make it less demanding, e.g. linking boring tasks such as cleaning or admin to compassionate care or other personal core value). Consider aspects of your own job and look at small adjustments that you could make to either the tasks, your relationships or the way you think about the tasks which could make your job less demanding.
- Reduce hindrance demands, where possible – Not every hindrance demand can be reduced (e.g. the number of people on a ward at any given moment may not be within your sphere of control) but consider any that can. Examples could be exploring shifts to minimise interference with non-work commitments, laying out of the admin/desk area to make the most efficient use of time, minimising daily hassles by exploring ways those infuriating tasks could be done differently. As with the job crafting above, these could be small changes, but you may also find that these changes could benefit your whole team.
- Seek out opportunities for challenge demands that allow for growth – Being able to use our skills and develop new ones is important for our self-esteem and work self-efficacy. Challenge demands can be on the job, such as assisting an experienced midwife with a particular technique you have not used before, or can be more formalised, such as training for a specialist role. When seeking out challenge demands it is important to consider what support you have to ensure success, so they do not become overly depleting.

When seeking out and protecting resources ask the following questions:

- Do you have all the physical things you need to do your job? Personal Protective Equipment, equipment for the tasks you need to do, etc. If not, what avenues are there to making sure you do?
- Do you have the social resources you need to do your job? For example, a formal or informal mentor, colleagues you are able to talk to or a work friend, non-work support network. It is also worth considering what type of support you need from them, as it will be different for each.
- Do you have the psychological resources you need to do your job? Consider the ways you cope with work, are they helpful/unhelpful? What thoughts do you have about work, are they helpful/unhelpful? Many of the other chapters in this book can help with exploring some of the psychological resources shown in the literature to protect against work stress such as self-awareness, proactive coping/goal setting, self-compassion, etc. Consider which ones may be useful for you.

When we are overloaded and stress/strain is prolonged, there is an increased risk of burnout. In the United States, there has been a move to make burnout a diagnosable clinical condition, but this is not the case elsewhere. In the United Kingdom, for example, someone with the symptoms of burnout may receive a diagnosis of clinical depression but the symptoms being experienced by individuals are often similar. Burnout is a term used a lot in everyday language, but it has three specific criteria to determine whether an individual is suffering from burnout; emotional exhaustion, depersonalisation and reduced personal accomplishment. Importantly for caring professions such as midwifery, two of the main symptoms (emotional exhaustion and depersonalisation) make compassion harder as people feel overwhelmingly tired with a sense of dread, irritation and an emotional detachment to the work being done. There has been much evidence generated in relation to burnout in midwifery populations, particularly since the launch of the Work Health and Emotional Lives of Midwives (WHELM) study (Hunter et al. 2019). Overall, managing the demands and resources at work outlined above, as far as possible, can help mitigate a potential loss of compassion. The following section focuses more specifically on ways we can maintain our compassion and its importance for healthcare.

MAINTAINING COMPASSION

Compassion has been defined as 'the combination of underpinning emotions (such as sympathy and empathy), with altruistic values, (particularly a desire to help others), which together motivate an individual to take action, which would ultimately be experienced as "care" by the recipient' (Kneafsey et al. 2016, p. 74).

Healthcare services may seem (ironically) like an uncompassionate place to work at times. Yet what might compassion in the healthcare workplace look like? In 2018, healthcare workers were asked to share their perceptions on what showed workplace compassion via a social media platform using the hashtag #ShowsWorkplace-Compassion (Clyne et al. 2018). The analysis showed that small acts of kindness, an embedded organisational culture of caring for one another and recognition of the emotional and physical impact of healthcare work were the most frequently mentioned characteristics of workplace compassion in healthcare.

More specifically, an organisational culture of speaking openly to learn from mistakes was cited as showing workplace compassion in this context as well as supporting staff to 'speak out safely'.

'Learning from mistakes instead of punishing #ShowsWorkplaceCompassion'.

No blame and no bullying leadership and management were also referred to as characteristics of workplace compassion.

'Meaningful action & education to identify & act on bullying #ShowsWorkplace-Compassion'.

Other comments captured on what shows workplace compassion included 'No belittling of staff' and 'No gossiping and no bullying' ... 'treat others as we would wish to be treated'.

Moreover, participants highlighted how 'Compassionate teams are key. Do we care about, value and respect everyone in the team?'

'Nurturing good people by valuing, respecting, rewarding them #ShowsWork-placeCompassion'. Evidently, 'Being trusted and being listened to is important' as 'If [staff] feel heard & empowered they'll treat others [the] same'.

Enjoying the workplace was also a characteristic of workplace compassion for some participants. Examples of this include 'Having fun at work important—#ShowsWorkplaceCompassion' and 'laughter... #ShowsWorkplaceCompassion'.

The use of caring language was referred to as demonstrating workplace compassion.

'Recognising the importance of language #ShowsWorkplaceCompassion... "we" "us" "colleagues" "people" not "you" "they" "staff" "human resources"'.

Personalised policies and procedures were seen as key to showing compassion in the workplace. One participant highlighted this by describing how 'my team were fab after the death of my husband' and another described how 'on the loss of his mum colleagues bought my husband a tree to remember her'.

Workplace compassion is described as generally as 'recognising what matters to one another'.

Small acts of kindness showing workplace compassion were described as 'asking how are you today especially to junior staff and a smile goes a long way' and 'A moment to make a cup of tea, to share a difficult time #ShowsWorkplaceCompassion'. Such acts were highlighted as 'making a big difference'.

Reflecting on the above, consider how compassionate your workplace is. How might you demonstrate compassion in the workplace?

As you can see from the contributions above, compassion is different to sympathy or empathy alone in that it factors in a desire to reduce suffering. Equally, being compassionate does not always mean just being nice; sometimes the most compassionate thing you can do is have the difficult conversation, create clear personal boundaries or state objections. Any of these actions can indeed be compassionate when they come from a place of reducing suffering, rather than from ego or self-preservation.

Why Is Maintaining Compassion Important?

Demonstrating compassion towards others and compassion towards one's self is associated with better mental well-being and loneliness across the adult lifespan, and physical well-being in younger adults (Lee et al. 2021). Compassion towards one's self or 'self-compassion' is a positive psychological strength which enables one to find purpose and meaning in one's life rather than simply pursuing pleasure and avoiding pain (Neff and Knox 2017). Self-compassion is particularly useful in moving past shame (Germer and Neff 2013). According to Neff (2003a, p. 89), self-compassion includes the following three elements:

1. Self-kindness – extending kindness and understanding to oneself rather than harsh judgement and self-criticism.
2. Common humanity – seeing one's experiences as part of the larger human experience rather than seeing them as separating and isolating.
3. Mindfulness – holding one's painful thoughts and feelings in balanced awareness rather than overidentifying with them.

Self-compassion has immense potential for helping people to thrive (Neff 2003a,b). Benefits include:

- Improved self-esteem
- Improved health
- Improved motivation
- Improved body image
- Improved interpersonal relationships

Below is one midwife's experience of surviving and thriving with compassion on the front line:

'At the start of the global pandemic, I contracted COVID-19 whilst working in the frontline and was very unwell for six weeks. Having worked in infectious diseases and later specialising in HIV midwifery, I knew numerous colleagues who also contracted the virus but sadly, consequently died. Whilst still unwell with COVID-19, my agency contract was terminated. Although this relieved the pressure I had to return to work, it left me feeling very bitter as I had contracted the virus whilst working. I was also angered about how easily managers can "discard" professionals that are deemed not to be of any benefit to the system.

Early in May 2020, I was feeling much better. In celebration of the Year of Nurse and Midwife, and to channel the anger I was feeling, I set myself a goal to raise the profile of midwives and nurses, and their global contribution to a global pandemic. I set out to interview student midwives and nurses, registered midwives and nurses, educators and leaders from around the world. Interviewing 380 colleagues across the globe left me truly inspired, many of whom have been collaborative, innovative and responsive to the populations they serve.

Unfortunately, a consequence of my initial COVID-19 infection has been Long-COVID. Although I initially felt better, I had several relapses and was eventually referred for further investigations and specialist help. Four years on, I am still challenged by Long-COVID and spend half of my week coaching colleagues who have been affected by Long-COVID too. As I learned to live with it, I have had to prioritise my health and be holistic in its management – physical, emotional, mental and spiritual. I urge everyone reading this to do the same! Self-care is not selfish and must be prioritised. Only when one looks after themselves are they better able to care for those in their care. It saddens me that many midwifery colleagues are burnt out and expected to provide excellent standards of care for women and birthing people, when they themselves do not feel cared for. My advice to colleagues is to plan to care for themselves first! How do you nurture yourself – physically, emotionally, mentally and spiritually? How do you nourish your body, soul, mind and spirit? Plan to do so on a daily basis.

It is also essential that one builds a support village – personal and professional. Who provides you with support at home and at work? Just like we would not wait for our car to break down before we check it, it is important to build and nurture your support systems so they can continue to support you through mentoring, coaching and supervision. If you do not have a coach or mentor, enlist the support of one now. Take time out to outline what support you need and how a coach and/ or mentor could support your growth and development.

My greatest learning is not just to survive but also thrive by truly loving yourself. Love for self will ensure that you show the same compassion you have for those in your care for yourself too. When last did you show yourself how loved you are? Take time out now to do so and keep doing that every single day! Do so first, not last, because you matter!'

Dr. Ruth Oshikanlu, RN, RM, RSCPHN, BSc, PGDip, PGDip, MSc, DUniv

How might you demonstrate compassion towards yourself and your colleagues in the workplace?

All I know is that my life is better when I assume that people are doing their best. It keeps me out of judgement and lets me focus on what is, and not what should or could be.

– Brené Brown

OPTIMISING SHIFT WORK

We know shift work is not good for our health. Shift work disrupts our circadian rhythms as we are required to be active when we would normally be sleeping which impacts on sleep quality and quantity, fatigue, stress and other mental health disorders, risk of heart attacks and gastrointestinal disorders (Harrington 2001). Our performance can also be affected, with poorer performance during night hours and a greater risk of accidents and other safety events for shift workers, especially at night (Harrington 2001). However, it is a necessary part of midwifery to ensure that support is available at all times of day. So, whilst the evidence for shift work does not look great, there are ways to minimise the impact and keep yourself healthy and support your well-being despite working shifts.

There are different shift patterns being used across the health sector and in different countries so there isn't a one size fits all approach for advice. However, if you are reading this and have responsibility for setting rotas and shift patterns there are things you can do to protect your staff. The number of hours per shift is less important than the direction in which those shifts rotate. The health and work-life balance outcomes for working an eight-hour shift as compared to a twelve-hour shift are pretty much similar (Smith et al. 1998), however twelve-hour shifts are often preferred as they give longer rest and recovery time (typically three to four days at the end of a batch of shifts). It is important to factor in the risk of running into overtime, as going beyond 12 hours impacts on fatigue and emotional exhaustion.

Some types of shift patterns or rotations are more damaging to the body than others. Shifts that rotate backwards (day, night, afternoon) can lead to poorer sleep quality and quantity, work performance and work-life interference compared to forward rotations (day, afternoon, night) (Shiffer et al. 2018). This is potentially due to the direction of the rotation limiting the time available for rest and recovery. In a similar vein, having a fast (three to four days) rather than slow (six to seven days upwards) rotation with at least three days for recovery after night shifts provides an optimum pattern.

In addition to setting shifts to rotate in a more favourable direction, giving staff more control over their shifts can also improve well-being. Doctors in an emergency department who were able to select the shifts they work using an annualised hours system (within a set of defined parameters to ensure fair distribution of weekend and night shifts) reported better well-being and work-life balance as they were able to fit their work around family commitments or social engagements (Teoh et al. 2023). Having a sense of control over the way that we work is negatively associated with stress/strain and so being able to select shifts around other commitments can provide a greater feeling of control over our work environment and therefore protect against potential stress. Blocking out days up to a year in advance allowed the doctors in the study to better plan personal and family matters, but they were placed under fewer demands than in the old, fixed shift system (i.e. needing to find shift cover or swaps).

If you work bank/agency/ad hoc shifts, you do have a greater degree of control over when you work but it is important to make these work for you both physically and in terms of fitting in with family life. The same points apply on forward rotations so when choosing which shifts to work, keep in mind the ways in which they rotate. Also ensure there is enough time for rest and recovery between shifts. The optimum is to have at least a three-day break after each batch of night shifts and aim to adopt a fast-rotating pattern. Plus, of course, the guidance below also applies to you; self-care when you are not working is as important as balancing the shifts you do work.

Even if you do not have control over the shifts you work, there are things you can do to optimise your health and well-being. Rest and recuperation between shifts are really important, so maximise time to do activities that allow you to re-energise (sleep, self-care, exercise) and protect your health when working on nights.

- **Sleep:** The amount of sleep we need varies from person to person but somewhere between 7 and 10 hours is optimal. When sleeping after night shifts, you want to trick your body into thinking it is night-time. Using blackout blinds or an eye-mask plus earplugs can help reduce the amount of sensory input. Avoid using any devices an hour before going to bed, which applies to both sleeping in the day or at night. The blue light interferes with our natural sleep patterns and can prevent you from falling asleep naturally. In addition to having better quality sleep when off shift, power naps of up to 20 min have been shown to reduce fatigue in midwifery staff (Teoh et al. 2023). Whilst it may seem impossible on busy days, if there is an opportunity (and support from your line manager) power naps during quiet times on shift may help manage tiredness.

- **Self-care:** Engage in activities that are restorative and these will differ from person to person. These should be activities that help you 'switch-off' from work mode: meditation, reading, taking baths, taking the dog for a walk, listening to music, gaming, socialising. Find out what works for you. Part of self-care is also ensuring what goes into your body is good for you; eating nutritious meals, staying hydrated, supplementing if needed, taking prescribed medication in the way it was prescribed. Sometimes it can be the avoidance of some activities that are depleting such as doomscrolling social media, drinking unhealthy levels of alcohol (or any alcohol at all after shifts if you need to sleep) or taking other substances.

- **Exercise:** Exercise can come under self-care but there are some key points with exercise that can help with recovery from shift working. Regular exercise can help improve sleep quality and quantity so building low-intensity exercise into your daily routine can help recover from shift working. The World Health Organisation guidance recommends at least 150 min of activity each week for health benefits (World Health Organisation 2020). This can be anything that raises your heart rate above resting for 20 min or more in one session, e.g. walking, swimming, dancing, cycling. But heavy exercise should be avoided before going to sleep as the neurotransmitters released during intense exercise (such as adrenalin) can prevent you from falling asleep. Save heavy exercise for after you have woken up, so either first thing in the morning or if working a night shift, before going to work.

- **On a night shift:** Eat a high-protein meal before going to work, take healthy snacks (nuts, fruit, houmous/guacamole with veggies, popcorn) to work with you and try to eat regularly throughout your shift. Stay hydrated and aim to drink at least a litre of water or diluted juice throughout your shift. Avoid caffeine in the last four hours of your shift to give you the best chance of falling asleep when you get home.

MIDWIFING OUTSIDE THE SYSTEM

As a student midwife, you will have been taught the magnificent art, science and philosophy of midwifery. Yet, unfortunately, these utopian visions may not always translate into reality as midwives bump up against counterintuitive systems and ideologies. Consequently, at times you may find yourself constrained as a midwife in reaching your true potential. For example, policies and guidelines may restrict your autonomy (e.g. see Small et al. 2022). Equally, the laws, systems and scope of practice for midwives in your own country may leave you frustratingly restricted. Whilst it will be important to remain within the law, united in tackling such wicked problems and solutions focused, you may also find yourself looking to practise midwifery independently or midwife outside the system. This can be a challenging thing to do in many ways, particularly where people are looking to birth in ways which may be deemed by the system to be unorthodox. Yet as I once heard the inordinately wise Franka Cadee say as president of the International Confederation of Midwives (ICM):

> Women don't 'opt' for outside guidance care. We [health systems] opt for guidelines that don't include the needs of all women.

There will be more from Franka later in the book. For this section, we have solicited the wisdom of Paul Golden on surviving and thriving in this context. Paul is a midwife working independently and in a variety of government hospitals around the world. Paul is also trained in law and mediation. He lectures on midwifery, law, human rights in childbirth globally and remains focused on the next generations and women's choices. In this section, Paul offers some important insights in surviving and thriving whilst midwifing outside the system:

'I am a global independent travelling midwife. How and why did this become me?

I'm a twin born at home and therefore understood home birth for twins is normal, yet many find themselves experiencing unnecessary medical interventions for perceived potential and often simply theoretical "risks" in a risk adverse culture. This applies to twin, breech and virtually all pregnancies and birth it is possible to find some "risk" that can appear to require intervention.

Yet when I saw birth in various settings such as smaller birth units then in different countries, I could see that risk was something often constructed and imposed by a system that is focused on fear rather than physiology.

I have worked in Aotearoa (New Zealand) since 1991, where around half the midwives are independent. There, a simple change in the law to allow women the choice of their lead maternity care provider shifted many women from family doctor to midwife led care.

If we all look at our motivation to be a midwife, we will often see events from our own experiences, whether that is being born or giving birth that will shape our decisions. My own mother had five children, all born within 5 years by the age of 25. She had little support having migrated to England from Ireland as a young teenager. She will have done the best she could yet suffered transgenerational trauma from her parents and their parents as impoverished Irish crofters. My mother was the ninth of nine children living in basic crofting conditions of a one room hut in County Tipperary Eire. These stressors and traumas would later play out in her parenting.

My motivation to be a midwife came from many areas in my life including my childhood. I probably wished to help other mothers not to be stressed like my own, and in part found maternal love an attractive energy that drew me to work with women. Then working in neonatal intensive care, I was often asked to be at a birth due to my apparently being "kind, calm and confident."

I returned from working in Sri Lanka (studying acupuncture) and remote rural Australia to the UK to study midwifery after working as a paediatric neonatal intensive care nurse.

The "training" was good and bad like the practices I saw around me. I moved to "Free-range midwifery."

What Is it to Birth and Provide Care Outside the System?

I am a travelling midwife. Travelling midwives are amongst us as they always have been. We provide care to women who want to birth their own way without state interference.

We will look at how they do this through my experiences.

I have been a midwife for over 30 years and always providing care "independently" (and working inside many hospitals large and small).

Ideally, I would collaborate with whoever the woman wishes. This may include the local hospital or medical staff, or doula and natural therapists. It may simply be with the woman and her family.

When a woman knows what she wants for her birth and pregnancy care this helps us to work together. It can work to simply know what she does not want, i.e. hospital birth. Yet I find this is the most useful question

What would you like ...
how do you see your birth?

This brings a focus on creating possibilities. Birth is like life, full of possibilities and opportunities. We are constantly learning, reflecting and building new networks of ideas and connections within ourselves and our communities.

If I am in a remote region, it is essential to know what the backup facilities are. Even in a city there will be choices and a variety of options that can be useful if a medical resource is required and agreed to by the woman.

My work has taken me primarily from New Zealand Aotearoa through Asia to the UK.

How Do the Laws and Regulation Affect the Midwives Outside the System?

In general, many developing countries are happy to have a midwife working there. Especially if they have registration in a "developed" country. However, this raises the questions about regulation. Some countries have none and others too much.

(continued)

(continued)

Over-regulation stifles creativity, breaches human rights and restricts choices in childbirth.

This latter point is simply covered by the Right to Private and Family Life (Article 8 of the United Nations Convention on Human Rights [UNCHR]) (and was upheld by the European Court of Human Rights [ECHR] in Ternovsky versus Hungary 2012).

A woman has the right to determine how and where to birth.

This includes for the woman to choose who to birth with, to choose her birth partner(s) including the midwife. Whether a country is obliged to provide childbirth choices to include homebirth is of some legal debate with inconsistent cases in the ECHR. However, it appears logical that countries must provide midwives for all options. We have a current case in the ECHR Amira Cerimagic versus Bosnia (this was part of a BBC documentary on Our World).

We have founded Human Rights Action in Childbirth that takes, educates, and advises on legal actions. The following hypothetical case studies may aid you to reflect on some of the complexities involved in both midwifing and birthing outside the system.

Case Study 1

A woman having her tenth baby at home following three caesarean sections might be considered "high risk" yet the risks (whatever they may be) are hers.

The parents take the responsibility for their decisions in life and with birth. This was brought home to them with the death of one twin at a home birth. However, they were articulate and adamant that their choices and right to "bodily autonomy" are essential to them and that prior traumatising abusive hospital "care" did cause harm to them and their baby. The risks of hospital birth were greater than home birth. Therefore, they prefer to make their own choices to birth outside the system at home with a trusted known midwife.

What Are Families Wanting from Their Midwife?

In my experience, the following appear to be the main requirements:

Calmness
Confidence
Kindness

Why Are These Elements Missing in Hospital Systems?

There are undoubtedly compassionate caring people working in the healthcare system. However, they are often not wholly allowed to respect individual thinking and choices when there are resource and ideology issues. Lack of staff, lack of time and lack of collaboration appear to be common in many hospital systems in my experience. When issues are raised there are generally failures with leadership to engage with either staff or consumers. Both are frequently threatened or feel threatened to comply. We can consider how this manifests by reading in the following reports among others:

Ockenden DC (2022) Final findings, conclusions, and essential actions from the Ockenden review of maternity services at Shrewsbury and Telford Hospital NHS Trust. Department of Health and Social Care, London. (https://www.gov.uk/government/publications/final-report-of-the-ockenden-review)

CBE, Bill Kirkup. "The Report of the Morecambe Bay Investigation". (2015). (https://assets.publishing.service.gov.uk/government/uploads/system/uploads/attachment_data/file/408480/47487_MBI_Accessible_v0.1.pdf)

Case Study 2

A woman whose partner died suddenly before the birth chose to birth at home away from the hospital because of:

(a) *trust in her body, her baby and the birth process*
(b) *distrust in the hospital that did not work in partnership with her or give informed choices*

The woman had direct experience of hospital staff acting in a rigid way. Being apparently "kind" in a manner that was full of inflexibility. This was described as "Killing with kindness."

She raised the insightful question:

"What is the point of professional registration if it stops a midwife caring for a woman's choices?"

Truly informed choices (and refusal) come from having options and alternatives to whatever is being offered. This includes simply declining or even simpler, not giving consent.

Case Study 3

A woman's labour was progressing perfectly, albeit not on a hospital schedule. Therefore, this woman was offered an augmentation of their labour with the use of oxytocin. This woman was a vulnerable migrant who arrived in the UK from Albania without a partner or any family support. I was her midwife. She simply refused, and as consent was not given, the hospital medical staff could and would not go ahead with any intervention.

This contrasts with other experiences particularly in Europe and Asia where there is less litigation, less human rights and less dignity or choices in childbirth.

(continued)

(continued)

This reaffirms the adage that

*"We only have the rights we stand up for
(And we only have the power we believe we have)"*

We concluded legal action may well stop some abuse in childbirth.

*"They only do what they do because they can
They won't if they can't"*

There are many criminal violations that happen that appear to be protected by the institution of the system which can be challenged, and like other institutions will no longer have this protection in the future.

For example, the institution of marriage protected a husband from allegations of rape until R versus R UKHL 1991. The institution of various religions protected abusive actions that are no longer protected. Therefore, the hospital institutions will, and are, losing their ability to protect against systemic abuse.

My work and life have taken me on a wonderful learning journey to places and people beyond my imagination from Tijuana in Mexico to Sri Lanka, Korea, Russia, China, India, Vietnam and so many places making connections with inspiring, loving people.

I have learned most from the mothers and babies and am constantly amazed at the capacity for love in simple actions like breastfeeding, or the doula, partner and family providing loving care to a woman in labour.

Our children were born simply at home by a mother who believed she could do it herself, so she did. Now our children say 'I can do it myself' to most situations in life. This is transgenerational empowerment.

I'm reminded of the verse from The Prophet Khalil Gibran

**All children live in the house of tomorrow,
a place we cannot visit
not even in our dreams**

I celebrate life and all the creative opportunities that come even from the abusive situations. Everything is an opportunity, and especially conflict.

Mediation and mediation studies and practice have reinforced the notion of our interconnectedness, including all those we disagree with as part of ourselves.

Now I tend to provide both clinical and legal skills to others through teaching and practical work. I'm a visiting lecturer and midwife globally. This requires me to be in balance and to notice my triggers and needs to truly be present including being present for the needs of others.

My earlier years with Tibetans in north India and exploring spiritual and philosophical pursuits appear to have paid great dividends as I enjoy a peaceful life wherever I am.

I wish all great self-compassion'.

Paul Golden. RM (NMC), RN (NMC), BA, PGCEA, PGLE, FDR.
You can access Paul's eBook 'Keeping Midwives Safe' here: (https://midwifemediator.gumroad.com/l/lwirg)

Further reading on the issues introduced by Paul can be found in the recommended resources section at the end of this book.

IN CONVERSATION (SALLY AND KAREN EXPLORE PERSONAL THOUGHTS AND EXPERIENCES ON MAINTENANCE OF OCCUPATIONAL HEALTH)

KM We have so many demands on our time as academics and often they conflict with each other. Our work with students often requires a reactive approach taking us away from the deep work of thinking and writing, such as for this book. How do the demands you have now as an academic compare to when you were in clinical practice and how have you learnt over the years to manage those demands?

SP The demands I have now are very different from those I had before. Clinical practice placed demands on me in the very immediate sense and I found it very difficult to plan ahead. This left me in a constant state of readiness I think, which was quite anxiety inducing at times, particularly as some actions (or non-actions) may result in significant harm or even death. Now in academia, I very much have to prioritise conflicting and perhaps more complex demands in terms of what is meaningful, what is necessary and what is desirable. I tend to prioritise what is meaningful, after ensuring that necessary tasks are completed at pace. Anything else desirable takes a back seat to what I find most meaningful in my work. It's the meaningful stuff that keeps me motivated.

KM Absolutely, having meaning and purpose are definitely important. For me, it is also important to have clear boundaries between work life and home life, and that I do activities outside of work that are important to my identity. My days off work are family time and I am really strict about not working at all on those days. I've always loved the water and so spending time each week either in the pool or the open water, and in the summer in the sea, is really restorative. As I spend a lot of time on the computer taking time to get away from a screen also helps. Whilst I do have my work emails on my phone, I have switched the notifications off so that I can control when I access them, rather than feeling like I need to respond each time it pings. I guess it is about reflecting on what works for you and what doesn't and how you build work into your life, and that can be different for each of us.

SP My life tends to flow between work and home. I enjoy being flexible about what I do and when. It is often when I am out walking that the 'Eureka' moments come. Equally, I can be sitting at my desk with writer's block on what I am trying to achieve. If I take a significant period of time off work, it takes me around a week to properly unwind and switch off. This is something I am working on. However, working is never a chore if you love what you do!

KM   Before I was an academic, I used to work shifts, not nights like midwives do, but earlies [early shifts e.g., 5.30 a.m.–2 p.m.] and lates [late shifts e.g., 3.30 p.m.–11 p.m.] and I often found it hard to get into a healthy routine. But one thing I found helped was to plan and prepare. I would plan my meals for the whole week on a Sunday and then prepare as much as I could in advance. That way there was less to think about when I was tired and prevented me reaching for the quick and easy microwave meal or takeaway. What tips can you recommend that helped you manage to stay healthy when you worked shifts?

SP   The thing I have observed about self-care in particular is that it's not collapsing in front of the TV with a pot of ice-cream, it's actually a lot of hard work. It is basically parenting yourself as an adult. That is pretty full on... 'Don't have that second slice of cake'! ... 'Don't stay indoors all day, get some fresh air!' ... 'Get to bed on time!' all of those things you hear parents say to their children, you actually have to say to yourself and do. It is not easy. Preparing meals is a good thing to do, but being strict about sleep and exercise is also key.

KM   Completely agree, but when we are stressed, it can affect the way we think and react to things, including looking after ourselves. How do you know when you are starting to get stressed? Has that changed over the years?

SP   As I grow older, I learn more and more about myself. I know when I am getting stressed because I start to wake up way too early (2–5 a.m.) and find my mind racing. My muscles will be very tense, and I will notice myself holding my breath for no apparent reason. This was far more pronounced when I was earlier in my career. I try not to make any big important decisions whilst this is happening. I have learnt to notice my thoughts and behaviours and let them pass. In prioritising and talking about my health I am also better able to step back and be more objective in situations I find stressful. It's a skill I wish I could give to my younger self.

KM   That is great self-awareness in action there. For me, I know I am a bit of a perfectionist but that also means that I can avoid doing things through a fear of failure. Stress can come from my own thoughts about myself and my work. Therefore, I have been working on self-compassion over the last few years and being more kind to myself. I am way more forgiving of others than I am of myself, and I am working on switching that narrative in my head. It is definitely still a work in progress but as long as I am still breathing, growth and learning to be a stronger version of me is always possible.

SP   I am not a perfectionist and I fail all the time! Maybe I am overconfident at times too. This used to be frustrating earlier in my career because I had all these amazing ideas (from my perspective) but nowhere to go with them. Nobody to nurture my enthusiasm. Now I have opportunities to test out all kinds of ideas, and whilst sometimes feedback from a critical friend or colleague can seem blunt at the time, it's all part of a journey in which you can only reach your goals if you keep moving forward.

Activity – Self-Assessment Risk Scale

Certain behaviours and feelings can be an indicator of when stress may be having an impact in our lives. The following tools are designed to give you a self-assessment as to whether you may be at risk of work stress or stress-related illness. It is important to note these are not diagnostic tools but designed to provide a degree of self-awareness and signposting to certain stress management activities.

In the last two weeks have you experienced any of the following (0 = less than usual, 1 = about the same as usual, 2 = more than usual, 3 = a lot more than usual)

Trouble sleeping	0	1	2	3
Feeling withdrawn	0	1	2	3
Feeling on edge or jittery	0	1	2	3
Eating more or making unhealthy food choices	0	1	2	3
Missing meals	0	1	2	3
Inappropriate emotional reactions or mood swings	0	1	2	3
Unexplained headaches or muscle aches	0	1	2	3
Intrusive thoughts	0	1	2	3
Difficulty concentrating	0	1	2	3
Crying	0	1	2	3
Drinking alcohol/using other substances	0	1	2	3
Feeling low	0	1	2	3
Worrying or feelings of anxiety	0	1	2	3
Compulsive or impulsive behaviour	0	1	2	3
Muscle tension/clenching jaw or fists	0	1	2	3
Making mistakes at work	0	1	2	3
Increased sickness absence	0	1	2	3
Digestive issues	0	1	2	3

Scores consistently in the 2's and 3's may indicate that you are experiencing stress symptoms. If you are concerned that stress is having a negative impact on your life, it is important to seek professional support via your GP, family doctor or other mental health organisation appropriate for where you live.

Stress management activities can help alleviate stress symptoms. The following are evidence-based techniques which have been shown to reduce stress symptoms. Different techniques work for different people so if you try something and it doesn't work for you, try something else.

Progressive Muscle Relaxation – This technique can be done by either sitting up or lying down. Starting at your toes, tense your muscles for 10 seconds and then relax, and then move up to your legs and repeat. Work methodically through your

(*continued*)

(*continued*)

body up to your facial muscles and then end with tensing your whole body for 10 seconds and then relax, sinking into your chair or mat.

Mindfulness – Mindfulness is simply the act of conscious awareness. It involves focussing on the present moment to reduce the mental time travel of ruminating on things that have happened or worrying about things that haven't happened yet (if at all). Take time in the day to observe the events and notice the sensations around you; sounds, colours, smells, tastes, temperature, touch, etc. Courses and classes with trained practitioners can be useful for those new to mindfulness and there are examples in the resources section at the end of the book.

Meditation – Some forms of mindfulness may also include meditation but there are also lots of other forms of mediation. Meditation is a practice to train the mind and body to bring about a sense of peace and calm. Many different religions have forms of meditation as part of their rituals, such as prayer, chanting, body movements, etc. If you follow a faith, engaging in the rituals associated with the practice of your faith can bring about a sense of calm, and secular meditation has similar effects when practiced regularly (Anisman 2014).

Cognitive Behavioural Therapy (CBT) – The aim of CBT is to challenge and replace maladaptive thinking and behaviour patterns with more realistic and helpful ones (Anisman 2014). Sometimes the thoughts we have about an event or stressor can compound the stress symptoms we feel (catastrophizing, all or nothing thinking, blame, etc.) and CBT helps us identify when that is the case and provide an alternative response. The limitation of CBT is that it takes time and personal investment in the activities and so when we feel acute stress pairing it with other activities can help with relief of immediate stress symptoms.

Exercise – Exercise can improve the way in which our bodies handle stress through the effect on neurotransmitters in the brain such as serotonin, dopamine and adrenalin. Aerobic exercise has the greatest evidence for alleviating stress symptoms which includes walking, jogging, swimming, cycling, dancing or organised sport with even short bouts of 10–15 min enough to make a difference (Jackson 2013).

Nature – There is a growing body of evidence to show that being around nature has benefits for reducing stress symptoms. This can be getting outside in a green space such as a park, or forest, or countryside but even being surrounded by house plants has positive effects (Capaldi et al. 2015). Blue spaces are also thought to have restorative effects with marine and freshwater environments shown to improve well-being markers (Gascon et al. 2017).

Whilst these techniques have been shown to help with stress symptoms, it is important to also understand the source of the stress. Some life events may cause expected but temporary feelings of stress and will naturally dissipate over time, for example grief, moving house, getting married, getting divorced, etc. Other sources of stress may be more long term unless something changes. Where possible, addressing the root cause of the stress is more effective than managing the symptoms we feel. In Chapter 4, we explore problem-solving and decision-making as a tool for addressing potential sources of stress that can be modified.

When it comes to work-related stress certain organisational hazards have been identified as having the potential to influence employee health and well-being. These management standards are:

- Demands – the amount and type of work we have to do and the environment in which we do it.
- Control – how much say we have over what work we do and how we do it.
- Support – encouragement and resources provided by the organisation, line manager and colleagues which help us do our job.
- Relationships – promotion of positive working relationships and dealing effectively with negative behaviours such as bullying.
- Role – the level to which people understand the roles they have and any conflict between different roles an individual may have.
- Change – How well any organisational change is communicated and handled.

The HSE in the UK have developed a risk assessment scale to assess the level of risk from each of the management standard. The full scale can be found on the HSE website (see the resources section at the end of the book for the full weblink). If you have a management role within your organisation it can be used to determine any areas which would benefit from being addressed to reduce the risk of stress in your staff. At an individual level the following questions can give you an indication of potential risk factors for you at work (0 = never, 1 = seldom, 2 = sometimes, 3 = often, 4 = always);

Demands

Different groups at work demand things from me that are hard to combine	0	1	2	3	4
I have unachievable deadlines	0	1	2	3	4
I have to work very intensively	0	1	2	3	4
I have to neglect some tasks because I have too much to do	0	1	2	3	4
I am unable to take sufficient breaks	0	1	2	3	4
I am pressured to work long hours	0	1	2	3	4
I have to work very fast	0	1	2	3	4
I have unrealistic time pressures	0	1	2	3	4

(Scores consistently within 3 and 4 may indicate excessive work demands which have the potential to lead to stress symptoms)

(continued)

(continued)

Control

I can decide when to take a break	0	1	2	3	4
I have a say in my own work speed	0	1	2	3	4
I have a choice in deciding what I do at work	0	1	2	3	4
I have a choice in deciding how I do my work	0	1	2	3	4
I have some say over the way I work	0	1	2	3	4
My working time can be flexible	0	1	2	3	4

(Scores consistently within 0 and 1 may indicate limited control over the work you do which has the potential to impact on stress symptoms)

Support

If work gets difficult my colleagues will help me	0	1	2	3	4
I am given supportive feedback on my work	0	1	2	3	4
I can rely on my line manager to help me out with a work problem	0	1	2	3	4
I get the help and support I need from my colleagues	0	1	2	3	4
I receive the respect at work that I deserve from my colleagues	0	1	2	3	4
I can talk to my line manager about issues at work	0	1	2	3	4
My colleagues are willing to listen to my work problems	0	1	2	3	4
I am supported through emotionally demanding work	0	1	2	3	4
My line manager encourages me at work	0	1	2	3	4

(Scores consistently within 0 and 1 may indicate limited support at work which has the potential to impact on stress symptoms. Note you may have different scores for items related to line manager versus those for colleagues and may reflect different but important sources of support at work)

Relationships

I am subjected to unkind words or behaviour at work	0	1	2	3	4
There is friction or anger between colleagues at work	0	1	2	3	4
I am subject to bullying at work	0	1	2	3	4
Relationships at work are strained	0	1	2	3	4

(Scores consistently within 3 and 4 may indicate negative relationships at work which may have an impact on stress symptoms)

Role

I am clear what is expected of me at work	0	1	2	3	4
I know how to go about getting my job done	0	1	2	3	4
I am clear what my duties and responsibilities are	0	1	2	3	4
I am clear about the goals and objectives for my department	0	1	2	3	4
I understand how my work fits into the aims of the organisation	0	1	2	3	4

(Scores consistently within 0 and 1 may indicate ambiguity over your role and job expectations which has the potential to impact on stress symptoms)

Change

I am able to question managers about change at work	0	1	2	3	4
Staff are always consulted about change at work	0	1	2	3	4
When changes are made, I am clear about how this will work in practice	0	1	2	3	4

(Scores consistently within 0 and 1 may indicate limited communication around organisational change which has the potential to impact on stress symptoms)

When completing this risk assessment for yourself, it is worth reflecting on any areas where there may be potential to action change for yourself or via your line manager. For example, having greater autonomy over the way you work is strongly linked to better well-being outcomes at work so there may be ways of increasing the amount of say you have at work. Some issues need to be tackled at an organisational level and so encouraging managers to take a temperature check of your team or organisation as a whole can start to effect wider change to improve the risk of stress more widely. (Adapted from source Health and Safety Management Standards Indicator Tool [HSE])

CHAPTER 4

Responding to Workplace Challenges

INTRO TO CHAPTER

You will note that throughout this book, we never refer to the term 'resilience' as being something required for survival in midwifery. Having emersed ourselves in several International Practitioner Health Summits, we now understand that whilst resilience may be required for both anticipated and unanticipated episodes in clinical practice, it should not be called upon to resolve wholly preventable episodes (e.g. bullying, incivility and short staffing pressures). Put simply, if you have someone punching you in the face, you don't need more resilience. You need them to stop punching you in the face. In the context of asking healthcare staff to foster more resilience in the face of growing and avoidable workplace challenges, one is essentially saying that the problem lies with one's lack of resilience, rather than the oppressive systems in which they work. This is fundamentally gaslighting and victim blaming, as the victim raising the concern is essentially blamed for their own demise. In this context, we respectfully pursue other avenues to survival and will continue to challenge the working conditions of midwives around the world. However, pushing for system change takes time and we need to find ways to survive in the system as it currently is in order to have the capacity to work towards the changes we want to see. Just as in an aeroplane the safety advice is to put your own oxygen mask on first before helping others with theirs, it is important we look after our own mental oxygen so we can start to support others with theirs.

In this chapter, we explore workplace challenges in the context of maladaptive coping, including problematic substance use. We then offer insights in relation to adaptive coping, decision-making and problem-solving. Lastly, we will leave you with tools for challenging unhelpful thinking patterns that may exacerbate stress symptoms.

Surviving and Thriving in Midwifery, First Edition. Sally Pezaro and Karen Maher.
© 2025 John Wiley & Sons Ltd. Published 2025 by John Wiley & Sons Ltd.

COPING WITH STRESSORS

When faced with challenging, stressful or traumatic situations we all seek out ways to cope either physically or psychologically. Coping is an internal, action-oriented effort to manage the demands of a stressful event (Lazarus and Folkman 1991). The way in which we cope with stressful events can be helpful (adaptive) or unhelpful (maladaptive) and is developed over the course of our lifetime. Sometimes the coping mechanisms we use may feel helpful initially but over time can either exacerbate the original issue (e.g. trying to placate a bully, taking administrative work home to do off shift) or cause additional issues (e.g. drinking alcohol to unwind after a hard day).

In the previous chapter, we explored demands at work. Work demands are a type of stressor or factor that can be perceived as causing an adverse stress reaction. However, the mere presence of a stressor/work demand does not automatically cause a stress response. People's reactions to the same stressor may vary a great deal due to the way they both appraise the demand and the behaviours they employ in order to cope with it. The stress-appraisal-coping triad (see Figure 4.1) highlights the interaction between the presence of a stressor/work demand, the individual's thoughts about the stressor/work demand and the coping strategies they employ to deal with the stressor/work demand. The way we think about a stressor will influence how much stress we feel, e.g. if you have been asked to attend a birth with complications you may view this as a challenge and opportunity to test your knowledge and skills and therefore have a positive stress reaction, or you may view it as a risk with the potential to go wrong which may bring about a negative stress response. The appraisal we have of the stressor may also influence the coping behaviours we use. For example, in the first scenario, where the complicated birth is viewed as a challenge you may take a problem-solving approach, refreshing your knowledge to plan for what might be needed during the delivery. However, in the second scenario, you may start to ruminate about potential negative outcomes and procrastinate about what needs to be done through fear of the outcomes. Engaging in these different coping behaviours will have an influence on the levels of stress felt, with the second scenario likely to induce higher levels of stress response potentially leading to psychological distress.

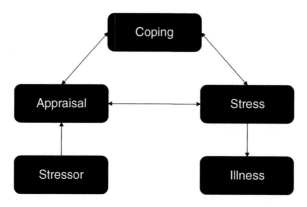

FIGURE 4.1   Stress-appraisal-coping triad. *Source*: Adapted from Lazarus and Folkman (1991).

Coping with stressors is a dynamic process and we adapt and adjust our behaviours based on feedback. Our appraisals of a stressor will influence the coping strategy we use, but our appraisal of the coping strategy will influence whether we continue with that strategy or try something else. The coping strategies we employ have been learned from early childhood through the feedback we get from our engagement with the environment and our caregivers. By adolescence, we have developed a toolkit of strategies, which for most of us will be broadly helpful in managing the demands we face (Wadsworth 2015). However, the strategies we employ may be helpful in some situations and unhelpful in others highlighting the dynamic nature and continued appraisal as part of the coping process.

Coping has been theorised as a style (a relatively stable dispositional factor of each of us) or as a strategy (a behaviour employed based on a response to situational factors) (Anisman 2014). The dynamic nature of coping behaviours suggests that it is likely to be an amalgamation of the two, we have our preferred behaviours to draw upon which we adapt dependent upon the situation. The coping methods available to us are broadly categorised into three areas: problem-focused, emotion-focused and avoidant. Problem-focused methods involve a cognitive process such as problem-solving or restructuring thinking about the stressor. Emotion-focused methods include a range of strategies such as emotional regulation, emotional suppression, rumination, blame or withdrawal. Avoidant methods include denial or disengagement. Generally, problem-focused coping is seen as helpful or adaptive and emotion-focused/avoidant coping as unhelpful or maladaptive, however this is a little simplistic and depends on how and why those behaviours are being used. For example, social support can be used adaptively to explore different options to deal with stress, or emotionally as a way of offloading problems, or avoidantly by being distracted with other activities. Likewise, regulating emotions (having a reasonable and proportional emotional response to the stressor) can be adaptive as it can allow for effective and honest communication, however emotional suppression/ dysregulation is maladaptive.

Adaptive coping involves healthy behaviours that help reduce the stress response. Key strategies outlined in the literature include:

- Active – problem-solving, seeking appropriate support, cognitive reframing.
- Accommodation – adjusting expectations (e.g. forgiveness or compromise).
- Emotional regulation – allowing a reasonable and proportional emotional reaction to the stressor.
- Behavioural – healthy physical behaviours to regulate stress response (e.g. exercise, meditation, talking with a friend).
- Cognitive – healthy mental activities to regulate stress response (e.g. seeking out positives, looking at the bigger picture).

Maladaptive coping involves behaviours that may temporarily alleviate the symptoms of stress, but because the underlying issues are not being dealt with any relief is only short-term. In some cases, e.g. substance use or self-harm, such behaviours can create longer term harm. Examples of maladaptive coping behaviours outlined in the literature are:

- Problematic substance use – use of alcohol, narcotics or prescription drugs to alleviate stress symptoms.
- Emotional dysregulation – either inappropriate or disproportional emotional reaction to the stressful situation. May be either under or over reaction (suppression or outburst).
- Rumination – running over the problem in your mind over and over, worrying.
- Blame – placing the fault of the problem in others and avoiding responsibility (other-blame), or holding all the responsibility (self-blame).
- Avoidance and distraction – ignoring the problem or pretending it doesn't exist or engaging in activities to forget about the problem.

The appraisal process is important in whether adaptive or maladaptive coping strategies are employed and are in response to the questions: *How stressful is this situation? How urgent is it? Do I have control?* Our responses to these questions may be different for different stressors and situations which means we may use different coping strategies for different stressful events. The following questions provide an indication of the coping strategies you generally use when dealing with stressful events. When you have completed the questions consider whether any of your responses are considered maladaptive.

Coping Strategies

Consider the following activities and indicate the degree to which you have engaged in them in response to stressful situations over recent weeks (0 – Never, 1 – Sometimes, 2 – Always).

1) I accepted that there was nothing I could do to change the situation   0   1   2

2) I made plans to overcome the problem   0   1   2

3) I told myself that other people have overcome problems like mine   0   1   2

4) I tried to distract myself from my troubles   0   1   2

5) I engaged in leisure activities I enjoy   0   1   2

6) I went over the problem in my mind over and over again   0   1   2

7) I made jokes or wisecracks about my problem   0   1   2

8) I talked to friends and family about my problem   0   1   2

9) I had emotional reactions (crying, anger, sadness)   0   1   2

10) I thought about who is responsible for my problem (other than me)   0   1   2

(continued)

(continued)

11) I thought about how I have brought my problem   0   1   2
on to myself

12) I tried to keep my feelings to myself   0   1   2

13) I asked for God's guidance   0   1   2

14) I fantasised about unreal resolutions to my problem   0   1   2
(revenge, winning the lottery, etc.)

15) I found comfort in my favourite food   0   1   2

16) I drank alcohol or took other substances to make me   0   1   2
feel better

1 = passive resignation, 2 = problem-solving, 3 = cognitive restructuring, 4 = avoidance, 5 = active distraction, 6 = rumination, 7 = humour, 8 = seeking social support, 9 = emotional expression, 10 = other-blame, 11 = self-blame, 12 = emotional containment, 13 = religion, 14 = wishful thinking, 15 = eating, 16 = substance use.

Which strategies do you employ the most frequently? It is important to note that some strategies can be both adaptive and maladaptive dependent upon the situation, so it is worth reflecting on how and why you use those strategies. For example, if there are demands at work causing stress going to the gym when you are not on shift as a distraction can be adaptive (active distraction), however if you have problems at home going to the gym is avoiding the problem rather than dealing with it then the same activity can be maladaptive. Emotional expression can be adaptive in the right situation (e.g. with a supportive friend or loved one) but maladaptive in others (e.g. in front of patients), whereas for emotional containment/suppression the opposite may be true in the same situations. This is where emotional regulation is an adaptive response and knowing when and where to express felt emotions in a safe way. Similarly, religion can be a source of comfort for many people in times of difficulty, however if this is engaged with passively (e.g. God will sort this out for me) it can lead to maladaptive behaviours such as avoidance rather than when engaged with actively (e.g. God will give me strength to overcome my problems) which can lead to problem-solving behaviours.

A little later on in this chapter, we explore ways to develop adaptive coping strategies and the exercises at the end of this chapter focus on cognitive restructuring of thoughts around stressors to be more helpful and active.

Scale adapted from Survey of Coping Profile Endorsement (SCOPE) (Matheson and Anisman 2003). Full scale available at (Anisman 2014, p. 68).

PROBLEMATIC SUBSTANCE USE

Substance use is one particular maladaptive coping mechanism that we have identified as having an impact on midwifery. The available literature on substance use in midwifery prior to our exploratory study in the United Kingdom was exceptionally limited

(Pezaro et al. 2020b) despite there being a wider acknowledgement that substance use in the healthcare sector is an issue requiring intervention, principally for physicians (Baldisseri 2007; Gerada 2021; Merlo et al. 2022). Studies in nursing populations suggest between 8% and 20% of nurses meet the criteria for problematic substance use and, given the similarities in work demands, it was reasonable to think that similar figures would apply in midwifery. However, we wanted to explore whether that was the case.

Our first study in 2020, collected data prior to the COVID-19 pandemic and found that of the 623 midwives who responded, 28% met the diagnostic criteria for problematic substance use (Pezaro et al. 2021a). Worryingly, of those 28% who met the diagnostic criteria only 11% indicated that they had attempted to seek help and 27% felt they should seek help but had not. Reasons cited for not seeking help included fear of repercussions (e.g. losing job/professional registration), shame and stigma, not knowing where to go or feeling there was nowhere to go for help, practicalities of getting the help (e.g. being too far away, not having time, etc.) or feeling like their usage was not a problem. This highlighted a large proportion of midwives who were attempting to survive at work whilst managing problematic substance use. Reassuringly, the vast majority of respondents had compassionate attitudes towards midwives who were impaired through substance use and, apart from a minority of oppositional attitudes, most felt that problematic substance use should be dealt with as a health concern rather than through punitive action. Unfortunately, minority voices feed into the shame and stigma those using substances feel, with respondents sharing shocking instances of public shaming and bullying type behaviour once substance use in a colleague has been identified. Many midwives spoke of the need to hide their usage so as not to meet the same fate as colleagues, which creates an additional burden as they attempt to carry on at work with, ostensibly, a health condition being untreated and concealed.

When we recollected data again in 2021 the number of midwives meeting the same benchmark was substantially higher at approximately 60%. The substance used most often, by a large margin, was alcohol followed by sedatives with smaller but not insignificant numbers of respondents indicating using recreational substances as a way of coping with work demands. With alcohol being a socially acceptable drug, it is unsurprising to see use of this particular substance increase in response to a significant increase in work and personal pressure or trauma. One of the mechanisms by which substances are suggested to help with work stress is through producing a stimulant effect thus regaining energy lost through work (Frone 2016). However, this effect is often short-lived. For example, alcohol induced sleep is less restful and restorative than natural sleep and over time can increase fatigue levels and other health consequences, which strengthens our argument for taking a health first approach to substance use.

One of the key findings from both studies was the lack of consistency regarding the way in which managers and employers dealt with substance usage cases. Some respondents shared stories of a supportive approach where individuals were able to get treatment and return to full duties once well, whereas others recall incidents of punitive action with police intervention and dismissal. By taking punitive action, skilled and experienced midwives are being needlessly lost from the profession in some cases. In addition, taking a person-centred approach to investigations can reduce 'avoidable employee harm' as well as reduce the amount of time lost from work, providing considerable financial savings to the organisation (Jones et al. 2023; Teoh et al. 2023). Of course, we appreciate that any criminal behaviour should be investigated in the appropriate manner, but we advocate that the default option should be to explore whether this behaviour is a result of a health condition rather than an act against probity, and if so, that person should be provided support for that health condition first and foremost.

In our survey, midwives shared deeply personal stories of how substance use had affected them, and we hope we have done them justice in the papers we subsequently published and that this is the beginning of a different approach to problematic substance use in midwives and healthcare professions more broadly. We were approached by a midwife from the United Kingdom, who has kindly offered to share her powerful real-world account of problematic alcohol use below.

Other People's Opinion of Me Is None of My Business

'What image comes to mind when you hear the word alcoholic?

Probably not what you, me or your colleagues look like, but in reality, addiction does not discriminate, it doesn't care who it affects or whose life it ruins. I don't like the word alcoholic, as both a professional and someone who has suffered with the inability to control their alcohol use. The stigma associated with the word makes it difficult for those of us who don't fit that stereotype to get the support we need.

I always had a "binge-drinker" lifestyle going out with my husband as well as drinking together in front of the telly on the weekends we were at home.

Drinking after a bad week, or a good one for that matter, was an escape from the mundane ritual of life without physically escaping it. But this was OK because it wasn't affecting my life. Or was it? I can't pinpoint where it became a problem or when I started drinking even if he wasn't, but I do know it really was a problem!

Drinking alcohol regularly or to excess is seen as a social norm. It's available in petrol stations, almost every shop and even in children's play areas. You just have to scroll through social media to see memes about alcohol, trivialising its misuse or as you leave work hearing someone say 'what a day, I'm having a drink tonight' validating that everyone else is doing it so it's OK.

And it is ok, until it's not OK anymore.

In 2018 I had a mental breakdown, I was a senior Midwife working in the community and like all of my colleagues I had a high workload, the team I was working in was a difficult team and there was a lot of pressure on me as the newcomer to improve working relationships, my relationship with my partner at the time was also falling apart by this point and I had two young children to juggle with work, one of whom has additional needs, with this on top of my mild depression and history of trauma it was a recipe for disaster.

I plunged into a pit of severe clinical depression and uncontrollable anxiety, having regular panic attacks and suicidal ideation, this is the point where a bottle of wine every night became my crutch, it soothed my anxiety and helped me sleep. The only problem was that very quickly it was no longer enough, one was no longer enough. In the evenings sitting on the sofa drinking the wine my anxiety was cured, it was working. The next day, however my anxiety intensified. Have you heard people jokingly refer to "hangxiety" (hangover-anxiety)? If you haven't experienced it, I can tell you it is VERY real.

My anxiety was unmanageable, I was calling into work sick, I was drinking more and drinking earlier in the day. I admitted to my manager the truth about my mental health and alcohol use. My head of midwifery spoke with me and advised I go off long-term sick, get the support I need and then return. WOW! This was amazing. I got my act together, I still suffered with anxiety and depression, but I was on new medication that seemed to be working...

I completed a phased return to work, finishing my last supernumerary shift I went home to return the following night for a night shift. I started to panic about the best way to sleep and take my medication, one of the medications I was on also acts as a sleeping tablet. I decided to try to stay awake and then sleep the next day. The next day I couldn't sleep even with the antidepressant, so I also took a sleeping tablet and set my alarm ready for my night shift.

Next thing I know it's two hours past my shift start time and my phone is ringing. I was too scared to answer. I had also received a message from the ward sister asking if I was ok. I explained in a message I had taken some medication and couldn't come in. I then had a panic attack, so I walked to the shop and bought bottles of wine. I drank away the anxiety until I passed out.

I woke up the following morning, my husband had taken the kids to school, he was angry, and I had a text from him telling me I better call work. The panic came flooding back. I still had wine left in the fridge so of course I started to drink it, that would help...

I had a knock at the door and a manager was on my doorstep, she had come to check on me. My colleagues were concerned for my welfare considering their knowledge of my mental health and alcohol use and were suspicious about the relationship with my partner at the time.

I admitted what had happened, they did a safeguarding referral for my children, discussed it with the head of Midwifery, spoke to my General Practitioner (GP) and arranged for a friend to collect me and take me to her house to keep me safe whilst I sobered up. My world was falling apart. A few days later I was advised to come in for my next shift as normal. Phew, they are still being supportive, I'm not sure why?

When I arrived at work, I was asked to attend a meeting before my shift. At this meeting I was suspended pending investigation. It was the worst feeling imaginable. I was given so much support that day in the meeting, my union representative and midwifery advocate were there. The midwifery advocate gave me a small token handmade gift to show me that everyone cared. I left work and returned home. I couldn't deal with the guilt, the shame and the fear.

I felt like I had let my colleagues down; I had let my children and my family down. Not because I didn't have respect for them. It was only a lack of respect for myself.

I spent the day crying, having panic attacks and trying to make sense of how I got here.

The next day I decided it was too much, so I bought a bottle of wine and took a whole packet of paracetamol. My husband couldn't get hold of me and came home; he realised what I had done and called an ambulance.

(continued)

(*continued*)

I was treated for paracetamol overdose in hospital. When I arrived home, I had the letter from the regulator. A few weeks later it was time to go to the regulator's fitness to practise board 300 miles away. It was terrifying whilst I was sitting there answering questions clutching onto the handmade gift given to me on the day I was suspended. It seemed like it was a solution-based process rather than a punitive one.

My suspension from work was lifted, I could return to work and I was determined not to mess it up. I completed all my training updates and orientation.

Then my husband and I suddenly separated. My life was falling apart again.

I held it together fairly well at first then before I knew it a glass of wine whilst the kids were at their dads became a bottle. I was calling in sick again, I wasn't eating, and I didn't care if I lived or died. I was drinking more, and more often. I handed in my notice at work as I knew that I wouldn't be able to keep my job anyway, I was too far down this pit of doom, time passed by and I had short periods of abstinence, my children were living with their dad although I was seeing them regularly when I could manage to stay sober enough.

The months passed and friends fell away, family were angry with me, my kids were not as loving towards me, and my ex-husband was furious.

As the months went on my alcohol use increased, I was regularly covered in bruises and feeling unwell all the time. It was only a matter of time before something bad happened.

I had a fall in my garden and sustained a head injury which led to an admission to hospital, I had a further fall and at some point, I had sustained a traumatic brain injury. I woke up in the Intensive Therapy Unit in a hospital with a specialist unit. I didn't want to be there, I self-discharged, getting a taxi home, my friends were informed I had left the hospital and were of course delighted to walk into my home, where I had somehow managed to climb through the window, to find me drinking! They had finally had enough and had to take a step away. I was later diagnosed with epilepsy due to the damage to my brain from the fall.

I was bored, I was heartbroken and I was lonely; friends were taking turns, coming to check on me each day but this was disrupting their own lives, work and family. I was wasting time scrolling through a dating site one day, I didn't want to date anyone, the dates I had been on were just to waste the rare time when I was childfree and sober. Someone I knew from a long time ago who I used to work near messaged me. We arranged to meet up, I was a mess, I was drunk and wanting to drink more, I was unsteady on my feet and emotional. This man took me to his house, helped me eat, gave me small sips of alcohol to stop me from withdrawing, helped me wash my hair, and tucked me into sleep. I now see that I am incredibly lucky, I was so vulnerable at that time. Anything could have happened to me. Luckily, he supported me over the following weeks to get the help I so desperately needed; I went to rehab.

After I left rehab, I started to think about returning to Midwifery. I went to work bank shifts at another provider before taking a role in the COVID-19 vaccination site. When this was coming to an end, I started to consider putting my personal experience to good use. I now work within the clinical team for the same substance misuse organisation that supported me. I have since become a prescriber. My understanding of addiction and substance misuse has come from my personal experience and from the people I was in treatment with. I made some really good friends in my time in treatment, unfortunately three of those friends have since died as a result of their addictions.

I attended a GP appointment recently where they asked me how often I have a drink containing alcohol, I replied, 'less than once a month' and I realised that's the first time in my life I have ever answered that question truthfully. Some people must never drink alcohol, some people can return to occasional binge drinking and be fine, some people can maintain safe alcohol levels. I think I have found my perfect recipe for recovery, enjoying the little things in life I used to take for granted, self-care and respect for my body by eating well and avoiding regular alcohol. I'm still smoking unfortunately, but it's in my plan to quit eventually. I may be wrong but for now it's working. Everyone who has struggled with substances faces the risk of returning to active addiction every day. It's terrifying, which is why most of the time it's easier to just choose my favourite sober treat, which is usually elderflower presse, not the stereotypical orange juice. I have control over alcohol after it had control over me for so long, probably a lot longer than I or anyone around me knew.

The turning point in my recovery that I will always hold was driving home and deciding I fancied a drink, it was raining, and I didn't want to get wet. Only a few years before I would have crawled over broken glass, naked, in the snow to get a drink from the shop (I didn't stop and buy the alcohol that day).

I am now working as an independent prescriber in substance misuse and as a bank midwife back where I was previously employed, it feels like home to me.

My (now) ex-husband and I are sharing care of our children, who are really happy and healthy, they seem to have forgiven me for being an absent parent.

My friends are back in my life and our friendships are being restored.

My family are so relieved and proud of me.

That Man that helped me when I was at rock bottom very quickly became my rock, best friend and later my partner. I became his wife in spring 2023.

My anxiety is well controlled, I don't suffer from depression, and I don't take medication for these anymore.

When I consider how my employer handled my situation, I can't fault how they did it. They were kind and compassionate, treating me as a person throughout.

I saw the reference a manager wrote to the regulator about my practice as a midwife. Highlighting that there were no concerns about my practice and only my health.

I see the kindness on my colleagues' faces when I tell them where I have been and some of my story when I return to the unit I had previously worked at to do bank midwifery.

Had the way I'd been treated been punitive rather than supportive I think it's likely I wouldn't be writing this today. I would likely still be very deep in active addiction or sadly no longer be here, leaving my children permanently without a mother, my granny without a granddaughter and my friends wishing I had just listened to them.

When I was discussing writing this, I questioned the impact it may have on me for sharing my story and then I remembered that other people's opinion of me is none of my business. When I started to realise this, I started to recover from my anxiety.

The only validation I need is from myself, for my colleagues to know that I am a capable prescriber and a capable midwife. My patients to see that I'm kind and compassionate as well as my partner, family, friends and children to see the love that I have for them.

(continued)

(continued)

I can't change other people's opinions, I can't change anything that's out of my control, I can only change how I react to it and that will not be by using it as an excuse to drink!

I am proud of my journey, I have been to rock bottom, I intend to never go there again and to support people in any way I can to prevent them from hitting their rock bottom. I urge anyone struggling with their mental health and/or substance misuse to reach out, find a way out before it's too late.

Reasons I used to find to drink alcohol to excess.

It's sunny
It's rainy
I had a good day
I had a bad day
It's my birthday
It's your birthday
It's the weekend
It's not the weekend
I'm happy
I'm sad
And so on ...
Reasons I now find not to drink to excess
I don't like hangovers, it's a waste of the day, I have wasted enough already
My kids
My Fiancé
My family
My mental health
My physical health
My career
I nearly died hitting my head and I don't want to risk another fall from intoxication'

Midwife from the United Kingdom

It is important to view substance use through the lens of compassion. The above story is a powerful one and highlights some of the key issues that arose in our own data. There are structural factors in midwifery that impact on usage and seeking support:

- Stigma, shame and bullying from colleagues can lead to the hiding of substance use perpetuating the issue and associated risks further through a sense of not having a way out.
- Fear for their jobs and the risks to professional registration also led to an inability to come forward for help. Many of the midwives in our study loved their job and being a midwife despite the demanding conditions they were working under and so the thought of losing their job was devastating.

- Policies being enacted subjectively meant that there were differences in the experiences of midwives engaged in substance use. There was a degree of luck involved as to whether the policy would be enacted compassionately with health in mind or punitively with performance management in mind and it often depended upon the opinions of the reporting manager.

We have met with some resistance in conducting this research including comments that we should not be bringing this issue to light as it tarnishes the reputation of midwifery. For us, the sweeping of substance use under the carpet and pretending it is not happening or taking punitive action against those found impaired has bigger risks to patient safety and quality of care than tackling the issue from a compassionate health first perspective. The midwife's story highlights the power of compassion in those first interactions with colleagues and managers, and how it can shape the direction of an individual's recovery. Midwives are human beings with human reactions to events the same as any other, and so should be afforded the same options when struggling as the rest of society. Midwives hiding impairment in an attempt to keep their jobs, whilst delivering perinatal care, risk safety incidents more often and more severely than if they were able to get support and have work adjusted until they were healthy enough to return. Not only does this reduce the risk to patients, but also keeps valuable, skilled and passionately engaged midwives in the profession for longer at a time of a severe retention crisis throughout the world. However, this requires a joined-up approach across all levels in healthcare organisations.

At the organisational level, there is a need for the creation and reinforcement of distinct drug and alcohol use policies which use supportive and compassionate health first pathways. Subjectivity in the interpretation of these policies should be removed through a clear decision-making tool for managers to apply which covers the variability in job roles across health services. Working with regulators in the development of these policies can ensure a consistent approach and ensure midwives are not dismissed prematurely and allow for the possibility of an individual to return to full duties once no longer impaired. With this in mind, it will also be important to stamp out any stigmatising behaviours such as naming and shaming or bullying, as these reinforce the perception of a punitive response and undo any potentially positive work at the policy level.

At the team level, line managers should ensure they feel competent and confident in dealing with substance use issues within their team using a health first approach. Training for the identification of impairment and what to do to support colleagues with problematic substance use should be offered to all staff.

At the individual level, there needs to be provision and treatment for staff with temporary work adjustment away from clinical care, if necessary. Employee Assistance Programmes (EAP) have shown good efficacy in other healthcare professions (Baldisseri 2007; Merlo et al. 2022) and similar programmes for midwives can allow for treatment and return to clinical practice. Fear of losing professional registration or their job creates a barrier to attending EAPs for substance use meaning they traditionally have a low take-up. Providing such programmes via anonymous media (app or web-based programmes) can mitigate this. Whilst these individuals may still be in clinical practice undetected, the risk to patient safety is offset compared to if they were not seeking help at all.

If you are worried about your own substance use:

- The first step is to identify whether your usage is problematic through considering the impact on yourself and those around you. In the resources section, we have included a link to a self-assessment tool you can use.
- Seek help in a safe way. Understanding your employer's policy on dealing with substance use behaviour may arm you with knowledge as to the best approach. Our research has highlighted that subjective interpretation of policies mean that not all employers treat substance use in a compassionate way and employ punitive measures where they may not be warranted. If you feel approaching your line manager or occupational health service is not a safe option for you, then anonymous support groups, such as Alcohol Anonymous or Narcotics Anonymous can provide initial steps towards getting help.
- Be aware that withdrawal from certain substances, such as over-the-counter pain medication or alcohol, can be dangerous if not monitored by a health professional. Before attempting to stop your usage, seek professional advice. Depending on your location, healthcare providers may have a duty to report substance use in midwives to regulators and so it is important you are aware of this risk when seeking advice.

If you are a manager or colleague worried about someone's substance use:

- Contact regulators for advice in designing local policies and procedures, particularly where they take a health first approach and will be supportive in providing guidance on how to navigate the next steps.
- Adopt non-punitive and supportive approaches as these may be most useful in promoting recovery and reducing risk where problematic substance use is a behavioural symptom of ill health. Our research has shown that onlookers in the same situation can be discouraged from seeking help themselves where punitive, rather than compassionate action is observed in response to such cases.
- Prioritise confidentiality to promote help-seeking and recovery, recognising problematic substance use as a behavioural symptom of ill health in the first instance.
- Actively deal with any naming, blaming and shaming actions from colleagues to shut down these behaviours as quickly as possible. These dissuade help-seeking and are harmful to recovery and professional reputations.

TOOLS FOR ADAPTIVE COPING

Adaptive coping involves dealing with stressors in a healthy way that allows for the protection of the health and well-being of yourself and others around you. The different approaches to coping have been outlined earlier in this chapter but what is important to outline here is that we can adjust the strategies we use when faced with stressors. Having a toolkit of coping strategies will give you the best chance of choosing a healthy coping behaviour over an unhealthy one.

Our coping strategies are learned behaviours, developed from childhood. Whilst we may have learned to cope automatically in ways that may be unhelpful, because they are learned behaviours it means we can learn new ways of coping that are more helpful. However, the first step is to understand when our coping mechanisms are unhelpful and maladaptive. The short questionnaire earlier in this chapter is a good place to start to understand your default coping strategies, the next step is to reflect on the impact of those strategies and whether they are being applied in the appropriate way for the situation.

Appraisals and beliefs play a large part in the way we cope with stress, and Shakespeare summed it up well in Hamlet when he wrote:

> *[T]here is nothing either good or bad, but thinking makes it so*
>
> (Hamlet II.ii)

The role of appraisals and beliefs about an issue can to a great extent explain why the same event can cause one person a great deal of stress and anguish, yet another person appears calm and unaffected. Many traditions and perspectives dating back thousands of years suggest that we can challenge the automatic beliefs and appraisals we have about life. Stoic philosophers understood we had the capacity to change our internal narrative through rational questioning of the thoughts we have to develop self-control over our response to life events. In a similar way, Buddhist philosophers propose that the suffering we experience is not due to the event/pain we feel but our thoughts about it, and by altering our relationship to the event we can reduce our suffering.

> *Pain in life is inevitable, but suffering is not. Pain is what the world does to you, suffering is what you do to yourself.*
>
> (Gautama Buddha)

One adaptive strategy to have in your toolkit is *cognitive restructuring*. This is the process of altering how we think about a stressful situation and identifying when thoughts we have about a situation are adding to our feelings of stress. Some automatic thoughts we have are irrational and don't stand up to scrutiny when interrogated further. Some common thinking errors include:

- Mind reading – inferring negative thoughts in others ('my colleague didn't say hello to me this morning. What have I done to upset them?')
- Magnifying – blowing events up out of proportion ('It is so awful that I didn't get my promotion, this is the worst day of my life'.)
- Personalisation – blaming ourselves for outcomes that are either wholly or not totally our fault ('I should have tried harder to give the families in my care the birth experience they wanted'.)

- Fortune-telling – predicting worse case scenarios with limited or no evidence ('What is the point in trying to put my change management project into practice, we never have enough staff, so it is just going to go wrong'.)

- All or nothing thinking – viewing events in extremes without any nuance or shades of grey ('Nobody ever listens to my ideas; I am just another cog in the midwifery wheel')

- Discounting the positive – framing any positive events as unimportant or down to luck ('My line manager is just being nice when they give positive feedback, my work isn't that good really'.)

- Phoneyism/imposterism – Fearing that others may find out we are not the person we show ourselves to be ('One day I will make a mistake and then everyone will know that I am not a good midwife'.)

- Demanding – having unrealistic expectations or rigid beliefs about events (should, musts, needs to, ought to, etc.) ('We should never be short staffed' or 'every day we ought to meet our targets'.)

The activity at the end of this chapter provides an opportunity to explore your thinking patterns and develop healthier ways of thinking about the same issue. Some alternative thinking skills include:

- Self-compassion – thinking about yourself in the same way you would about your best friend or loved one. Rather than being critical of yourself when things don't go according to plan, step back and reflect on the event more accurately ('I needed help using a piece of equipment today but that doesn't mean I am useless as I now know how to use it next time'.)

- Relative thinking – Rather than thinking in extremes introduce shades of grey or a middle ground. ('Sometimes we are short staffed, and the team are doing an acceptable job within the resources we have'.)

- Seek evidence – Rather than attempting to mind read or fortune tell, seek out evidence so you can draw a more informed conclusion to the event. ('My colleague didn't say hello this morning, I'll ask them if they are ok'.)

- Demagnification – Instead of blowing events up out of proportion, take a more rational or detached view of events. ('I didn't get my promotion which is a shame, but I can try again next year'.)

- Look at the bigger picture – rather than focusing on immediate emotions, reflect on how important this event is likely to be in the next day/week/month/year/10 years. ('This report feels important now but in a year's time, we will be in a wholly different place within our team')

- Keep emotions in check – Instead of using emotions as evidence of negative outcomes, remind yourself that emotions do not always mean you are under threat or there is the likelihood of a bad outcome ('I am feeling anxious about doing this procedure but that doesn't mean it won't go according to plan, I am just feeling an emotion'.)

Social support is another excellent coping resource for your toolkit, and it works on multiple fronts. The role of social support will differ depending on the situation, person or stressor and can be used for emotional support, information gathering, guidance, reassurance/confidence building, detachment from the stressor or problem-solving. Firstly, on an emotional level connecting with others can diffuse negative emotions and enhance positive ones and can protect against stress developing into depression (Anisman 2014). Secondly, social support can act as a distraction from the stressor allowing the stress response to dissipate so we have lower levels of those fight or flight chemicals in our bodies (Heinrichs et al. 2003). And thirdly, social support can promote active coping through seeking advice and talking through action plans to reduce the impact of the stressor. However, the quality of social support is also important with trust and relatedness valuable for how well social support influences our stress levels. This is why support groups for people going through similar experiences have success through support coming from 'someone who understands'. It is also important to note that not all social support is positive as sometimes it can allow for maladaptive behaviours (e.g. peer encouragement or acceptance of substance use, using social activities as a way of avoiding dealing with an issue, gossip which reinforces thinking errors). So, it pays to be mindful and reflective about the ways in which social support is guiding your coping behaviours. Where optimally implemented, Schwartz rounds® can provide staff with a safe, reflective, and confidential space to talk and support one another too (Maben et al. 2021).

When seeking social support:

- Cultivate relationships at work through finding your community of midwives (see Chapter 2).
- Get to know people at work beyond their work identity. Make regular conversation when making tea or in down times to get to know about peoples' lives outside of work and share parts of your own life that you are comfortable with. By making regular but incremental social conversation we can strengthen our relationships and build trust.
- Develop friendships and social networks outside of work. If you don't already have a network of people joining clubs (sports clubs, reading groups, crafting groups, etc.) can be great places to meet like-minded people.
- If you have a particular issue with which you would like support, you may find a support group that already exists either in-person or online. Various social media platforms host a wide range of groups for people with specific health conditions, parents of children with additional needs, neurodivergent conditions and much more. These often provide a safe(r) space to ask advice or seek emotional support from people who have been through the same thing.

Understanding the root cause of the stressor may uncover that stress symptoms are related to a personal boundary being crossed or taking on too much through a desire to be helpful and please others. The activity at the end of Chapter 5 provides the opportunity to explore *boundary setting* and scripting responses when a personal boundary has been violated. Part of these boundaries is about how we use our time and being able to say no to people is an important coping strategy to prevent us from being over-loaded. Some tasks are essential and therefore expected as part of our role, however others may be discretionary, going above our expectations. Sometimes we take on these discretionary tasks because we want to help others, or they are exciting or interesting to us, or we think they may help with our career progression. However, the more we take on the more thinly we spread our time which can impact on the quality of the tasks we do or whether we can achieve them at all. Reflection and self-awareness can help us understand whether we have the capacity to take additional work on when asked and where our desire to say yes may be coming from. Ways to say no can include:

- If the request is coming from a colleague and you do not have time in your workload to do the task, be honest but avoid getting into details. 'Normally I would love to help but my workload at the moment means that I just don't have the time'.
- If from your line manager and your workload is at capacity highlight the demands on your time and ask what tasks to prioritise. 'I can see that you would like me to do X task but I currently have A, B and C tasks which are taking all of my time. Which are the priorities and which can I push back?'
- If the request is something you are interested in or useful for your career development that you would like to do but currently don't have the capacity, seek to keep the door open for future opportunities. 'Thank you for thinking of me and I am really interested in getting involved in a project like this. My work-load at the moment means I am not able to commit just now but please keep me in mind for future work'.

Sometimes the root cause of the stressor may not be able to be actively dealt with until a later point and so having healthy coping strategies to deal with the stress symp-toms can be useful until the cause can be acted upon. Adaptive *behavioural* activities such as engaging in hobbies, exercise, meditation, socialising with friends can provide a distraction from the stressor but it is important to recognise when these are a healthy distraction, when no active approaches can be taken or when they are avoidant behav-iour. Activities that bring you joy will be much easier to go to than ones that don't so don't push yourself to go for a run if you don't like running just because exercise is shown to be a good stress relief; find a form of exercise that makes you smile and you are more likely to use it when stress feelings arise.

As well as the adaptive coping strategies above, one particular coping strategy which has consistent evidence in the literature as being related to positive outcomes for stress symptoms and performance is problem-solving. So much so that we felt it deserved a section all of its own.

PROBLEM-SOLVING AND DECISION-MAKING

Generally, in decision-making you can avoid problems by planning for and managing risks alongside challenging information and encouraging healthy debate. You can also avoid feeling paralysed in decision-making by validating the outcomes of decisions already made and embracing continual learning. Additionally, to assist in guiding your decision-making, Drucker (1967) presents the following model for making what they call '*The effective decision*'. This model includes the following steps:

1. Categorising and defining the problem
2. Gathering information
3. Identifying consequences and considering alternatives
4. Weighing the evidence
5. Choosing among alternatives
6. Acting
7. Reviewing decisions

This may serve as a useful and logical framework for you and your teams to sequentially abide by in developing and improving high-quality services for example. Nevertheless, sometimes action can be seen as being more advantageous than inaction. Yet doubt can be a source of valuable insight. Kahneman et al. (2011) offer a few helpful questions to ask yourself before you leap into any big decision:

1. To check for self-interested biases (*where we take individual credit for positive outcomes, but blame outside factors for negative ones*), ask: is there any reason to suspect the team making the recommendation is motivated by self-interest?
2. To check for the affect heuristic (*where benefits are exaggerated and risks are minimised for preferred options*), ask: has the team fallen in love with its own proposal?
3. To check for Groupthink (*where the desire for group consensus overpowers common sense alternatives*), ask: were there dissenting opinions within the team? Were they explored adequately?
4. To check for saliency bias (*where we favour only particularly remarkable information*), ask: could the judgement be overly influenced by an analogy to a memorable success?
5. To check for confirmation bias (*where we prefer evidence which confirms our hypothesis over that which opposes it*), ask: are credible alternatives included along with the recommendation?
6. To check for availability bias (*where we only rely on examples immediately available to us*), ask: if you had to make this decision again in a year's time, what information would you want, and can you get more of it now?
7. To check for anchoring bias (*where we are swayed towards our preferred outcomes/estimates*), ask: do you know where the numbers came from? Can there be ... unsubstantiated numbers? ... Extrapolation from history? ... A motivation to use a certain anchor?
8. To check for the Halo effect (*where views are formed from first impressions only*), ask: is the team assuming that a person, organisation or approach that is successful in one area will be just as successful in another?

9. To check for sunk cost fallacy (*where actions are continued purely because they have had resources invested*), endowment effect (*where we value something higher simply because we own it*) ask: are the recommenders overly attached to a history of past decisions?

10. To check for overconfidence, planning fallacy, optimistic biases, competitor neglect ask: is the base case overly optimistic?

11. To check for disaster neglect (*where we fail to consider the worst-case scenario in going ahead with a plan*), ask: is the worst case bad enough?

12. To check for loss aversion (*where we consider the pain of losing to be more powerful than the pleasure of gaining*), ask: is the recommending team being overly cautious?

Other top tips to avoid bias traps include:

- Reviewing proposals with extra care, especially for overoptimism
- Rigorously apply quality control checklists
- Imagine that the worst has happened, and consider the possible causes
- Rebuild the case with an outsider view
- Reconsider the problem as if you were new to the job
- Solicit opposing views, discreetly if necessary
- Ask for more analogies, and rigorously analyse their similarity to the current situation
- Seek additional comparable examples
- Request additional options

IN CONVERSATION (SALLY AND KAREN EXPLORE PERSONAL EXPERIENCES OF RESPONDING TO WORKPLACE CHALLENGES)

KM I have no doubt that midwifery is full of challenges every day. Are there any notable challenges that you have come up against in your career?

SP Absolutely. In my clinical career, I struggled to 'fit in' where my progressive ideas clashed with more conservative midwives. Over twelve years ago now, I also found myself struggling with two undiagnosed health conditions whilst working in clinical practice. A lack of insight into what these health conditions were and how to manage them appropriately meant that problematic substance use and other symptoms, triggered by traumatic incidents at work took hold. It was a terrifying time, which ultimately ended in my mental and physical health breaking down. My fitness to practise was impaired and I had to focus on how to manage both health conditions effectively following formal diagnoses.

KM That does sound like a difficult time not just for you but also for those living through it with you.

SP   I was really shaken. I was also shocked at how my own poor health could result in such a lack of insight – a total inability to recognise what was happening to me or the need to seek help. It took approximately two-years for me to learn how to manage my newly diagnosed health conditions properly. Moving into new environments with new colleagues helped.

KM   That is a long time to be struggling. What was the turning point for seeking help? Was it a single incident that triggered that decision or gradual insight over a period of time?

SP   At the time, I didn't understand what was happening to me. I couldn't articulate it and felt paralysed. I was also displaying some symptoms in which I didn't recognise myself. Ultimately this is what prompted intervention. The relief in finally opening up was immense, but I didn't start to develop insight into the situation until I started engaging with treatments, physicians, consultants, experts and therapists. My recovery and the development of insight were made harder by gossip and punitive responses. I lost my job too. What happened at the time would not have occurred *but for* my ill health, but that didn't feel relevant or even considered by some in the profession. On the contrary, the extensive regulatory investigation that followed led to conclusions which did focus on my health. Working with new groups of people who lifted me up during this healing time also allowed me to shine in ways I hadn't considered before. I started to see what I was capable of and what I could achieve in the profession for the first time as my health began to improve and I moved into other areas of practice.

KM   It sounds like you were treated as a whole person rather than just the acts which led to the investigation, which is exactly what we need to happen. We don't always see it at the time, but our darkest moments can bring about important personal growth. What has happened since then?

SP   It feels so good now to be in a workplace where I can thrive and enjoy good health again. I still feel like I am playing catch up on the time I lost through ill health and feeling a sense of being held back from where I could have been. There is so much I want to achieve. I continue to manage my health conditions every day, but I needed to go where I was celebrated, so I returned to midwifery practice in academia and research instead. I now use my own experiences to help others learn and grow, and to inform midwifery workforce and well-being research. It's why I do the work I do now.

KM   How about on a personal level? What has changed about the way you approach challenges now compared to earlier in your career?

SP   I talk to people about my health more now and listen when people advise me to take time out. I also have a toolkit of options for managing my health, and I am far more reflective about what I spend my time doing and what I prioritise. There will always be people who will never 'get' you, and that's OK. I now see more clearly than ever the need for compassion and kindness, both to oneself and others. This ultimately liberates me to live in the kind of world I want to live in, and work in the kind of profession I want to work in.

Activity – Tools for Challenging Thinking Patterns

Practising Gratitude

Negative experiences stick in our minds much more easily than positive ones which means we can often miss the good in life. Practising gratitude can force us to take notice of the positive things that happen, no matter how small and over time they become easier to spot. Regular gratitude practice has shown to help us reduce stress levels, have fewer negative thoughts and improve altruism and helping behaviours.

Practising gratitude is simply about being thankful for your life, the people and things within it and the experiences it brings. On days when things seem particularly bleak, that can be difficult but not impossible. Look for things that perhaps you do automatically that wouldn't ordinarily think about such as 'I am grateful for the clean water that comes from my tap so I can wash, cook and drink to keep myself healthy'. If you have had a challenging day at work and you are stuck ruminating over what went wrong or negative events, seek out the positives that may come from the event, e.g. 'I am grateful for the aggressive patient showing me how calm and strong I can be under pressure' or 'I am grateful for my colleague taking the time to show me how to record patient notes so that I can do my job to the best of my ability'. This isn't about pretending the negative event didn't happen or minimising its effects, but more about helping yourself move out of negative thinking patterns so that you are able to move forward in a positive way.

These are a couple of ways you can bring regular gratitude into your life:

- Write a gratitude diary – Before bed write down up to 10 things you are grateful for each day. These can be big or small. If you can't do 10 straight away build up to it over a couple of weeks. Start with one on the first day, two on the second and so on. The important thing is to build a habit.

- Take gratitude moments – At different times of the day take a moment to think about what you are grateful for right now. You can set a reminder for a regular time each day or just take random moments. Right now, for example I am grateful for the spring sunshine so I can work with the door open and listen to the birds while I type.

- Thank others – If someone does something that you are grateful for, let them know. Not only does it make them feel good, but it also makes us feel good. Some cultures find this easier than others but even if you feel awkward, if it is a genuine thank you, give it a go; what is the worst that can happen?

ABCDE Model

The ABCDE model is a tool from cognitive behavioural therapy (CBT) and rational emotive behavioural therapy (REBT) (Ellis and Ellis 2019) designed to help us spot unhelpful/irrational thinking patterns and provide alternatives that are more helpful/rational. Table 4.1 is made up of five columns. Starting with column A and moving rightwards across the table, complete each of the sections for something that causes you to react in a stressful way.

TABLE 4.1 ABCDE model worksheet.

Activating event	Beliefs about the event	Consequences of those beliefs	Disputing beliefs	Exchanging beliefs
The triggering event that causes stress reaction	The thoughts and beliefs you hold about that event	Internal and external behaviours created by those beliefs (e.g. avoidant behaviour, maladaptive coping, self-chastisement, rumination)	Challenge your beliefs, are they rational, what else could be involved?	Exchange unhelpful beliefs for more helpful, rational and balanced ones.

Source: adapted from http://happiertherapy.com.

CHAPTER 5

Thriving in Interpersonal Relationships at Work

INTRO TO CHAPTER

Working with colleagues can be tough, yet interprofessional relationships can make or break the workplace experience, particularly in how you are able to thrive (or not). In this chapter, we introduce evidence-based ideas on how you can enable your team to thrive, by building on inclusivity, psychological safety and trust. We also offer ways in which you might successfully resolve conflict and manage workplace incivility, through challenging inappropriate behaviours. Lastly, within this chapter, we walk you through effective boundary setting to help protect your well-being through the balancing of time and energy needs.

ENABLING YOUR TEAM TO THRIVE

In Chapter 2, we explored the need for your multidisciplinary community to thrive. But how do we make this happen? According to Salas et al. (2005), a well-functioning healthcare team requires five key dimensions:

- Team leadership
  - Ability to direct and coordinate the activities of other team members; assess team performance; assign tasks; develop team knowledge, skills and abilities; motivate team members; plan; organise and establish a positive atmosphere.

Surviving and Thriving in Midwifery, First Edition. Sally Pezaro and Karen Maher.
© 2025 John Wiley & Sons Ltd. Published 2025 by John Wiley & Sons Ltd.

- Mutual performance monitoring
  - The ability to develop common understandings of the team environment and apply appropriate task strategies to accurately monitor teammate performance.
- Backup behaviour
  - Ability to anticipate other team members' needs through accurate knowledge about their responsibilities. This includes the ability to shift workload among members to achieve balance during high periods of workload or pressure.
- Adaptability
  - Ability to adjust strategies based on information gathered from the environment using backup behaviour and reallocation of intrateam resources. Altering a course of action or team repertoire in response to changing conditions (internal or external).
- Team orientation
  - Propensity to take other's behaviour into account during group interaction and the belief in the importance of team goals over individual members' goals.

To be effective, these dimensions must be underpinned by:

- Mutual trust
  - The shared belief that team members will perform their roles and protect the interests of their teammates.
- Shared mental models
  - An organising knowledge structure of the relationships among the task the team is engaged in and how the team members will interact.
- Closed loop communication
  - The exchange of information between a sender and a receiver irrespective of the medium.

In reality, we can all probably think back to a time when trust was broken (or perceived to be broken) within a team, or where shared mental models were not always communicated or fully understood. In enabling your team to thrive, it will be important to reflect outwardly and inwardly upon whether these key dimensions are being met or, if not, could be worked towards. If we think about how some of these key dimensions could be achieved, we can also note the skills and tasks required to turn these visions into practice. How might you develop these key dimensions in your teams? And how might any barriers to developing them be overcome?

Explicit awareness that disparities and bias exist and can lead to differential treatment in clinical settings also distinguishes high-performing perinatal services from low-performing ones (Howell et al. 2022). In Section 5.3, we will explore how the benefits of equality, diversity and inclusion may be realised.

EQUALITY, DIVERSITY AND INCLUSION

In Chapter 1, we explored some of the ways in which midwifery may overcome gender inequalities through the dismantling of harmful and patriarchal gender binaries, rooted in colonialism. Yet for some years I (Sally) have also had the privilege of bestowing Mary Seacole Awards upon aspiring and ambitious midwives (and nurses) to undertake specific healthcare projects and activities to the benefit and improvement of the health outcomes of people from diverse Black and minoritised ethnic (BME) communities. The Mary Seacole Awards provide an opportunity for individuals to be recognised for their outstanding work in the BME community, perhaps better described as being 'global majority' communities. The awards were funded by Health Education England and awarded in association with the Royal College of Midwives, the Royal College of Nursing, UNISON and Unite with support from NHS Employers. The programme is now being run by the Mary Seacole Trust and the Florence Nightingale Foundation, and I still enjoy mentoring scholars through this programme and seeing what amazing work they continue to deliver every day.

A former Mary Seacole Scholar, Sarah Chitongo, conducted a hugely significant piece of qualitative research on midwives' insights in relation to the common barriers in providing effective perinatal care to those from minoritised ethnic groups with 'high-risk' pregnancies (Chitongo et al. 2022). Racism and unconscious bias underpin many of the findings presented. Communication was a key barrier to care. Minoritised groups were often reportedly not listened to, and where translation services were required, they were often unavailable or insufficient. A lack of continuity of care/carer was also identified as a barrier to global majority birthing people receiving high quality care. This was compounded by policies relating to one's immigration status and the need to move location or pay for healthcare in some cases. Ultimately, poor health literacy and/or competing social demands often meant that the wider social determinants of health acted as a barrier to high quality care for this community.

Co-created community hubs and orientation services may improve access to more effective perinatal care for Black and Brown people and promote knowledge exchange. Considering the racism which underpinned these findings, there must be more focus on robust anti-racism interventions, including the decolonisation of services. Midwives' well-being and education must also be prioritised in this area. Further, the safe provision of continuity of care/carer models may enable issues to be identified earlier, as trusting relationships are built throughout the pregnancy. As some midwives were expected to act as translators alongside their midwifery duties, the provision of bespoke translation services requires urgent attention. Overall, the barriers illuminated in this study illuminate how important work in the area of equality, diversity and inclusion is, and how change may be realised. The NHS Race and Health Observatory (www.nhsrho.org) works to identify and tackle ethnic inequalities in health and care by facilitating research, making health policy recommendations and enabling long-term transformational change. On a global level, the World Health Organization is also working to address racial discrimination (World Health Organisation 2022b). There is much work to be done.

In pursuit of equality diversity and inclusion, it is important to avoid putting people into single categories. Instead, we must begin to look at things in depth. This includes colleagues as well as service users. Viewing things from an intersectionality perspective may enable us to address wicked problems in relation to inequalities with more clarity. This is because inequities are never the result of single, distinct factors (e.g. sexual orientation, disability, gender). Rather according to Hankivsky (2014), they are the outcome of intersections of different social locations, power relations and experiences.

PSYCHOLOGICAL SAFETY AND TRUST

When working in teams, such as in midwifery, there is an interdependence between the team members; the actions, behaviours and performance of one team member directly influence the actions, behaviours and performance of the other members. In midwifery, you will need to use your discretion consistently throughout your work to make decisions and actions and the greater the feeling of trust from your leader and other team members, the more innovative and novel we can be in those decisions and actions. Psychological safety is a concept that originates from organisational psychology and refers to the perception individuals have about taking interpersonal risks within a group or within an organisation. The concept centres around the shared belief in a team that you are able to make decisions, express ideas and concerns, and admit mistakes without fear of negative consequences (Edmondson 1999). It is permission for candour and an understanding that work is a learning experience.

One of the leading researchers in psychological safety is Professor Amy Edmondson, an academic at Harvard Business School. In her original research, Edmondson (1996) found that in hospitals, contrary to expectations, effective teams made more errors than less effective teams. She hypothesised that this was because effective teams were more likely to admit mistakes because they felt safe to do so. Within healthcare, the ability to report errors and near-misses is crucial for patient safety through the learning that comes from them and so when teams feel safe to share errors, they are more likely to engage in behaviours conducive to learning. Rather than these errors having a detrimental effect on performance and patient outcomes, the teams with higher levels of psychological safety performed better through better diagnosis of, and dealing with, problems leading to improved patient outcomes.

It is important to note that psychological safety is not about being nice, or necessarily feeling comfortable with your team, as sometimes there are difficult conversations to be had to ensure effective learning takes place. Psychological safety is being able to have those difficult conversations without fear of personal attack or negative interpersonal outcomes, such as being ostracised. It is a common understanding within the team members about the overall goal of the team and an openness to novel ideas and behaviours.

Within any organisation there are certain factors, or antecedents, that contribute to a psychologically safe environment. These help to create a climate where individuals feel safe to express themselves, take risks, collaborate effectively and report errors and failures. In the literature, these antecedents are clustered around supportive leadership behaviour, relationship networks, the characteristics of the team and individual/team difference (Newman et al. 2017). Some of the specific factors include:

- **Trust and respect**: Trust and respect are fundamental building blocks for psychological safety. When people trust their colleagues and their leaders, and believe that their contributions are respected, they are more likely to feel psychologically safe.
- **Supportive leadership**: Leaders are important for setting the climate for psychological safety through modelling the behaviour they expect in their teams. By providing support and guidance through open communication they set the tone for the team and/or organisation.

- **Clear expectations**: Having clear and well-defined expectations within the team helps individuals understand their roles and responsibilities, reducing ambiguity and increasing psychological safety.
- **Inclusive culture**: Cultivating an inclusive culture where diverse perspectives and backgrounds are celebrated and respected promotes psychological safety. When team members feel their unique experiences and identities are acknowledged and valued, they are more likely to feel safe.
- **Learning orientation**: A learning-oriented culture sees mistakes and failures as opportunities for growth rather than reasons for punishment. When a learning orientation is encouraged, individuals are more likely to feel safe to take risks and try out new ideas.
- **Resources and training**: Making sure that team members have all the necessary physical resources and skills to perform their roles can boost self-efficacy and reduce feelings of insecurity.
- **Empowerment**: Giving individuals autonomy and decisional latitude within their roles can help them feel more in control and enhance confidence in their abilities.
- **Recognition and reward**: Recognising and rewarding contributions and achievements can reinforce a sense of value within the organisation. Rewarding effort not just when things go well can help cultivate a learning orientation.

However, creating a psychologically safe environment is an art rather than a science. Whether you are in a leadership position or a team member, aim to model the behaviour you want to see such as showing humility, open communication, active listening. These behaviours can become contagious within the team. If you hold leadership responsibilities establish norms for how failure and mistakes are handled (predictability and fairness), look for the learning, encourage constructive conflict but shut down personal conflict quickly and celebrate the wins, however small.

Psychological safety within the workplace can lead to a wide range of positive outcomes, both for the individual and the organisation as a whole. These can contribute to a healthier and more productive work environment. A review of the literature (Newman et al. 2017) highlights that psychological safety is related to:

- **Increased communication, knowledge sharing and voice behaviours**: Psychological safety encourages open communication and so team members are more likely to work together effectively, share information and support one another to achieve common goals. Team members are also more likely to point out mistakes in other members or supervisors, more likely to raise a disagreement and give candid feedback.
- **Increased learning behaviour**: Psychological safety has been related to greater learning behaviours following failure, both at the individual and team level.
- **Increased performance, innovation and creativity**: The increased learning behaviours have an indirect effect on performance through enhanced creativity, problem-solving and innovation. Not only is performance improved at the individual level, but psychological safety within teams has been shown to have a positive effect on wider organisational performance.

- **Employee attitudes**: Psychological safety has a positive effect on individuals' work-related attitudes such as organisational commitment (how committed they are to working for their organisation), work engagement (how absorbed, energised and dedicated they are to their work) and overall job satisfaction. These attitudes have a knock effect on turnover, whereby teams with high levels of psychological safety have lower levels of turnover, indicating that psychological safety could be a key concept to help address the midwifery retention crisis.

Whilst the discussion here around psychological safety suggests it is nothing but a good thing with huge potential benefits for the individual and the organisation, it is important to add a caveat, particularly when it comes to intercultural working. Much of the research in this area has been carried out in Western, individualist cultures (United States, Europe, Australia) and so there is a gap in knowledge around psychological safety in collectivist cultures. Many collectivist cultures may have a social penalty for speaking out and strong perceptions of hierarchy. Therefore, it is important to understand the diversity and cultural make-up of your team when expecting them to engage in behaviours linked to psychological safety and effective conflict resolution.

SUCCESSFUL CONFLICT RESOLUTION

Below is a real-life account of how one midwife survived and thrived in the face of conflict between medical and midwifery professionals in Qatar:

'Mummy as I'm called (due to being named after my grandmother) "I want you to pursue a career in Nursing and Midwifery, so my legacy remains when I pass on. You are my eldest daughter; therefore, you must step into my shoes." These are the words by my mother which still echo with me.

I grew up in an environment where being a nurse or a midwife was not a well-paid job, however, so much of inner satisfaction is gained through gratitude from families when you care for them throughout the pregnancy continuum.

My mother has a small care facility for pregnant women in Sierra Leone where I started working with her as a teenager. I remember growing up, pregnant women and their families will arrive with farming (crops, vegetables, rice, etc.) just to reward my mum for the nursing and midwifery care they received. Most of the girls born were named after her in the small town that we lived and where she practised. I saw her practice independently and autonomously which was difficult for me to comprehend because I assumed this was the role of doctors to deliver babies back then. It is worthy to note, however, throughout that period, she had no maternal death – she will proactively make referrals when there are deviations from the expected pregnancy trajectory. This is what attracted me to midwifery there upon I decided to pursue it passionately as a career as so wished by mum.

Not long after my State Registered Nursing training, I relocated to the United Kingdom where I worked for five years as a registered nurse before enrolling for the midwifery course

(continued)

(continued)

at City University London – as this had always been my dream. One would ask why it took that long. In a nutshell, I had to wait for immigration clearance, which happened one Friday (when I received the letter in the post), the next Monday I was in the lecture room starting my midwifery education. That was how eager and determined I was to pursue a career in midwifery – I believed this was my calling as predicted by my beloved mum.

Following my qualification as a Registered Midwife in the United Kingdom, I joined The Royal London Hospital in Whitechapel London, England. Working as a qualified midwife gave me so much pride and confidence. It reminded me so much of my mum. Thankfully, I was afforded autonomy to assess pregnant women including women in labour and postnatal women, developing, and executing care plans. I would only escalate cases when there are deviations from the normal. I worked in a team from diverse backgrounds with varied experience which was a positive influence for me. I had peers whose expertise were a step or two ahead of me. I understood that and would tap into their vast experience. This helped me to constantly update my skills and practice to ensure care for women is delivered using the best available evidence. This was indeed rewarding for me.

Practising in the United Kingdom as a midwife for eight years became my "comfort zone." I came to realise this when I relocated to the Middle East where care is completely obstetric led and different from the United Kingdom and Sierra Leone. To say I was shocked about what midwifery looks like in the Middle East is an understatement. To have managed to work in Qatar after stepping out of my comfort zone for the past five years is what I refer to as "survival of the fittest." Initially it felt as if I have been dumped in a lion's den – there were few registered midwives, no existing midwifery led model of care, medicalisation of childbirth and everything about maternity was obstetric led. Although during the recruitment process, I was informed that the role entails developing a midwifery led model of care, I didn't envisage the true picture or reality of things. It appeared as if there was no light at the end of the tunnel and I found myself in a very strange environment.

As someone who is very passionate about midwifery, I had to reflect on the best way forward. Women and health professionals were not familiar with the term midwifery, it is the medical profession that has gained respect and recognition. I observed outdated practices in the clinical area, less than 5% of the workforce within the obstetrics and gynaecology department are registered midwives, the concept of normality (physiological birth without intervention) was not evident and evidence-based practice was only in theory. It was an environment that felt you could not thrive with midwifery led care. My journey began as a Clinical Midwife Specialist (CMS), a clinical role that had little or no voice when it comes to operational and strategic decisions. I came to realise through the grapevine that it is very difficult to implement changes in the organisation if you are not in an operational role. I was not going to allow the status quo of midwifery to prevail. I was very much determined to be part of the history of change. This set me on the path to go for the Director of Nursing/Midwifery (DoNM) role when the position became vacant, albeit initially in an acting capacity but thereafter I successfully interviewed and was appointed as the substantive post holder. This now affords me the opportunity to influence strategic and operational decisions on midwifery among others.

During my role as a CMS, I advocated and developed group antenatal education sessions and vaginal birth after caesarean section clinic (VBAC) counselling sessions for women. The clinic provided evidence-based information to women that will empower them to make informed decisions about their pregnancy. This was the starting point for me. I have put forward a few midwifery proposals but unfortunately it has been delayed or declined for varied reasons. As a passionate midwife working in an obstetric led environment, I am constantly seeking innovative ways to improve service delivery as well as engage with stakeholders to embark on new programmes or projects, albeit one at a time. Some of the plans in the pipeline are multi-year projects. I also developed a divisional strategic plan that aligned with the organisation's women and newborn transformational plan and the National Health Strategy second priority focus which is healthy women leading to healthy pregnancies. I am proud to say within three years we have managed to accomplish 50% of the plan, 20% are ongoing activities and 30% yet to start or delayed due to the pandemic. Some highlights of achievements so far include:

- *A senior Registered Midwife (I) leading the service*
- *Developed a divisional strategic plan and a robust governance structure for the women and newborn division.*
- *In addition to the two existing midwives that were in post when I started, 15 more registered midwives and an additional CMS employed and currently in post*
- *Successful establishment of group antenatal education and VBAC clinics*
- *Commenced community outreach programmes on the role and benefits of midwifery care (put on hold due to the pandemic)*
- *Rolled out a community postnatal homecare service from the tertiary facility for women post LSCS and high-risk cases*
- *Established an infant feeding committee working towards the accreditation of a Baby Friendly Hospital Initiative (BFHI).*
- *Successfully implemented and now sustaining an early ambulation project for women 8–12 hours post LSCS from 6% to 100% within a year of commencing the project*
- *Supported the CMS in post in establishing a midwifery led antenatal clinic for low-risk women two days a week including developing an upskilling program for all midwives in post.*
- *Established a multidisciplinary (MDT) committee where issues are discussed, and midwifery care advocated for*
- *Developed a monthly pectoral spotlight for the division, highlighting indicators for midwifery, e.g. reducing episiotomy and caesarean section rates*

The above initiatives (key deliverables of the strategic plan developed) represent modest progress made so far considering these never existed. Having worked in countries where midwifery is recognised, it is natural to find it a challenge to work in a

(continued)

(continued)

predominantly obstetric led environment but equally comforting to know I have thrived and survived thus far. I am determined to keep pushing for reforms and evidence-based practice. I know I will be in the history of midwifery care in Qatar when it eventually comes to fruition. Giving up is not an option. I take the stumbling blocks as a learning curve to help women achieve healthy pregnancies leading to the best childbirth and postnatal experience'.

Mariama Lilei Feika, MSc, BSc (Hons), RN, RM, Director of Nursing & Midwifery, Al Khor Hospital – Hamad Medical Corporation, Qatar

MANAGING AND CHALLENGING WORKPLACE INCIVILITY

Internationally, midwives experience various types of work-related psychological distress. In particular, dysfunctional working cultures do not allow midwives or the midwifery profession to thrive, as midwives remain persistently concerned about workplace aggression, incivility and bullying (Pezaro et al. 2016). Workplace incivility is becoming an increasing threat to workplace productivity, absenteeism, motivation, staff retention and workplace well-being. The way in which we treat people, and each other matters. Bullying does not go unnoticed by service users (Pezaro et al. 2018a). It costs lives and money, as well as putting patients and the public at risk (Capper et al. 2021; Kline and Lewis 2019). Consequently, alongside strategies designed to reduce such incivilities, it will be important (unfortunately) to be able to manage and challenge these in the workplace.

Civilised behaviour does not include destroying other people, and so intrigue clearly lies in what might make people engage in uncivil behaviours in the first place. Within midwifery (a profession highly dominated by females), Tall Poppy Syndrome (TPS) has been introduced as a framework to explain how women in the workplace interact with other women they perceive as superior to them in some way (Peeters 2004). The 'Tall Poppy', is an Australian cultural expression referring to those who exemplify exceptional skills or admirable qualities. In TPS, those who interact with tall poppies often attempt to demean, destroy, or bring the 'tall poppy' down professionally in some way. But why?

People throw rocks at things that shine

– Taylor Swift

Envy, female competition, snap judgements and misperceptions are all directly related to TPS. Indeed, when people are unsure of themselves, lack confidence or lack relevant information about others, their perceptions become typically biased or distorted (Goffman 1959). In Mancl and Penington's (2011) work, 'envious others' are also termed 'poppy clippers', whose communicative behaviours can be subtle and indirect, and reflected via both nonverbal (e.g. not paying attention, giving the 'evil eye', not listening, not respecting you, but looking and judging-in-a-split-second') and verbal (e.g. gossip and 'backbiting') messages.

Some behaviours (e.g. rudeness and eye-rolling) may be passive, where the perpetrator may not even be aware of how they affect others negatively. Yet other extreme behaviours may be dysfunctional (e.g. causing intentional harm or discomfort to an individual – for example, through humiliation or shaming) or deviant (e.g. causing intentional harm to colleagues' safety [physical/psychological]). According to Roter (2018), these types of behaviours are motivated by something that addresses the need of an individual or individuals, in particular. As well as needing to manage and challenge such behaviours, victims may also need the tools to explore forgiveness in pursuit of the maintenance of their own psychological well-being. We will cover such forgiveness tools in Chapter 6. We also explore in Chapter 6 the escalation of concerns, which may similarly be useful in escalating concerns of this nature in practice.

It may be useful as a victim to understand that those with lower levels of emotional intelligence are more likely to display incivility in the workplace (Loi et al. 2021). Feelings of shame and guilt may also cause some people to aggress, whilst those who are more able and willing to take responsibility for their own actions and avoid blaming others are less likely to engage in incivility (Stuewig et al. 2010).

In our own research, we have established that midwives can resort to 'naming, blaming and shaming' those who transgress their own moral frameworks as a sanction of disapproval (Pezaro et al. 2022b). Such naming, blaming and shaming really have no place or value in midwifery, and may arise through feeling a misguided need to morally gatekeep the midwifery profession. Such behaviours reflect high expectations of moral integrity, which many describe as 'Doing the "*right thing*" even when no one is watching'. However, morality is socially constructed and so what may be moral for one, maybe immoral for another (as seen through conflicting views within religion, national law, political beliefs, etc.). Thus, in pursuit of levelling moral high grounds, it may instead be more practical and psychologically enriching to assume the position that everyone is doing the best they can at any given time, and perhaps even fighting a personal battle you know nothing about.

When confronted with a challenging colleague, to adopt a learning (instead of a blame based) mindset, knowing you don't have all the facts, try the following as suggested by Delizonna (2017):

- State the problematic behaviour or outcome as an observation, and use factual, neutral language. For example, 'In the past two months there's been a noticeable drop in your participation during meetings and progress appears to be slowing on your project'.
- Engage them in an exploration. For example, 'I imagine there are multiple factors at play. Perhaps we could uncover what they are together?'
- Ask for solutions. The people who are responsible for creating a problem often hold the keys to solving it. That's why a positive outcome typically depends on their input and buy-in. Ask directly, 'What do you think needs to happen here?' Or 'What would be your ideal scenario?'
- Finally ask: 'How could I support you?'

In addition to this, it may be useful to challenge behaviours by letting someone know how to get the best out of you. For example, try to finish the following sentence

'I tend to work best when ...'. If we can articulate how we need to be treated to thrive, we give those engaged in incivility the tools to change tact.

In addressing workplace incivility, it is important to establish psychologically and socially safe workplace cultures ('the way we do things around here'). We have alluded to this through previous chapters and have discussed psychologically and socially safe environments as something Sally needs to thrive as a midwife. A psychosocial safety climate (PSC) is defined as 'policies, practices and procedures for the protection of worker psychological health and safety' (Dollard and Bakker 2010, p. 580). It comprises four major principles:

1. senior management support and commitment to issues that affect employees' psychological health
2. management priority in resolving issues about psychological health and safety
3. organisational communication with employees about matters that affect psychological health and safety
4. participation and involvement by workers in issues on psychological health and safety

Whilst these organisational commitments will be crucial in promoting psychological safety in the workplace, we can all contribute to redefining what acceptable behaviour looks like in the workplace. This does not have to be done in a confrontational way, as a little humour may be all that's needed in diffusing situations or nudging a change in behaviour. Nevertheless, when bullying remains a problem, we can offer the following suggestions:

1. Maintain accurate records – A clear record of evidence will be key if you decide to take a complaint further
2. Keep to the facts to remain credible
3. Avoid retribution or vigilantism – The best revenge is personal happiness and success
4. Use independent volunteer networks (e.g. charities specialising in confidential counselling)
5. Access occupational health services where possible
6. Seek advice from Trade Unions
7. Stating the impact of the behaviour(s) and calling it out as unacceptable may be enough to resolve the issue – Do this with a witness if possible
8. Practise being confident and assertive in your body language
9. If you are a bystander or witness to bullying, your actions may alert the perpetrator to their bullying behaviours and others' reaction to it – create social peer pressure where possible to reset cultures and behaviours – highlight that 'this is not the way we do things here'
10. Validate the experiences of anyone who confides in you that they are being bullied – They may feel confused and will need someone with an open mind to listen

It is also important that we all monitor our own behaviours in pursuit of psychologically safe workplaces. The following questions are adapted from those posed by Rayner et al. (2002). Can you answer them positively?

- Are you aware of how you come across to your colleagues, students, staff, superiors?
- Do you ask for feedback on your behaviour in the workplace?
- Do you pay attention to your own emotions in the workplace?
- Does your body language always reflect what you are saying?
- Do you initiate or join in with jokes made at the expense of other people?

Below is an example of how workplace incivility relating to one midwife's 'direct entry' training status resulted in a stress response. Despite the challenges faced, you will read how this midwife continues to survive and thrive.

'I emigrated from the United Kingdom to Australia in 2001 and had been offered my dream job working as a midwife in a busy Metropolitan hospital in Western Australia. But when I arrived, my qualification as a Bachelor of Midwifery (Direct Entry) graduate was not recognised by Western Australia. I was only the second Direct Entry midwife to work in Western Australia, and rather than be defeated, I looked for ways to overcome this problem. I was advised to undertake a Registered Nurse programme of study to be able to work as a midwife in Australia. But I didn't want to be a nurse; I was a midwife. I found a better solution myself, by obtaining registration as a midwife in New Zealand, then getting trans-mutual recognition through the Nursing and Midwifery Board of New South Wales in Australia. I was then able to register as a midwife in Western Australia. This process was time consuming and so frustrating – yet I had good support from the hospital who wanted to employ me and midwives working in education who wanted to change the thinking about midwifery education in Australia. I knew I would not give up.

Finally, in 2002, I started working at a large metropolitan hospital near Perth in Western Australia, and I was contracted to work as a rotational midwife on the labour and birth suite (which was my favourite midwifery environment after qualifying as a midwife), and a postnatal ward. I looked at the roster on the birth suite and saw that after my name the initials (DE) were written. I immediately knew that I was being labelled as a Direct Entry midwife and could not understand why. I had not met with this kind of discrimination in the United Kingdom. I began questioning why it was necessary to label my training – I was working in a maternity hospital with no general patients – surely a midwife is a midwife regardless of training. I know some people began to think I was "challenging," but I was determined that there should not be any discrimination and questioned this practice until it was finally removed and not used again. I later found out that only one midwife had objected to midwives who did not have a nursing qualification as well and had instigated this process on the labour and birth suite.

(continued)

(continued)

I had been working six weeks as a midwife in Western Australia and was actually working on a postnatal ward when one of the midwives asked me if I was OK and if I could lift my arms. My right eye was watering but I was so busy that day that I had not had time to think about it. I didn't understand why she was asking me that and she told me to go and look in a mirror. I did, and the right side of my face had drooped. I realised my colleague thought I was having a stroke. The manager put me into a taxi and sent me to an emergency department at another hospital, where it was discovered that I had developed Bell's Palsy. I saw a consultant in the emergency department, who explained how the condition occurs and asked me if I had been under any stress. And in that moment, I realised I had been under a huge amount of stress trying to do the job I loved. But I was determined that this would also not defeat me, and I bought some eye patches (as my right eye would not close) and went back to work four days later. My speech was still difficult because I had a right-sided mouth droop, and I became known as the pirate midwife – and several years later I saw a lady in the supermarket (who I did not remember), and she said, "Oh hello – do you remember me? I remember you; you were the pirate midwife who delivered my baby!"

I had an appointment with a consultant a couple of weeks following the Bell's Palsy diagnosis and he wanted to stitch my eye closed to prevent damage to the eye as it would not close. But I had conducted my own research into the condition, and I had read a paper that talked about using plastic under an eye patch to retain moisture in the eye that would not close. I told him I wanted to try a method I had read about. He said OK, but he would monitor the eye and gave me some special eye drops to help keep it moist. So, I cut up a series of plastic shopping bags into eye-sized squares (they were given for free to pack shopping into at supermarkets at that time) and wore one under my eye patch. I continued to work and soon I seemed to become very accepted by both women and colleagues. After three weeks my mouth droop had nearly disappeared, and eight weeks later I was able to close my eye and the eye patch was no longer required.

I have encountered many challenges in my midwifery career, both clinically and academically, but the beginning of my clinical midwifery role in Australia was a difficult time. But I am a determined woman, and I pick my battles to fight. My midwifery career was central to my being – and I was determined to fight for it'.

Professor Sadie Geraghty, RM, PhD
Head of Discipline (Midwifery), Faculty of Medicine, Nursing,
Midwifery and Health Sciences
The University of Notre Dame Australia

Further sources of support on managing incivility can be found in the additional resources section at the end of this book.

IN CONVERSATION (SALLY AND KAREN EXPLORE PERSONAL THOUGHTS ON INTERPERSONAL RELATIONS AT WORK)

KM Sally, have you experienced conflict or difficult relationships at work when practising as a midwife?

SP I certainly had colleagues speaking to me very inhumanely in clinical practice more than once. It was a bit of a shock when it occurred. Jarring because it was so unexpected and inappropriate. It is easy to ruminate about how you would have responded if you could go back in time and experience the event again. I wish I'd had responses prepared at the time.

KM Well, hindsight gives us 20:20 vision.

SP Also, when I was unwell, I naively thought that colleagues would want to learn from what happened to me and support me in my recovery and subsequent return to practice, particularly as we were all working in the field of care. Yet when I was at rock bottom, it felt like some colleagues' behaviours were targeted to actively destroy me both professionally and personally. But at the time I needed compassion and support, not retribution. I had to adhere to and listen to the decisions, diagnoses and treatment plans administered to me at the time in order to get better and return to practice – If I was to thrive, I couldn't heed any negativity.

At the end of the regulatory investigation into my case, the facts and conclusions were heard entirely in private because they related to my health. This is one of the reasons why I am unable to discuss details. My experiences of trauma also mean that much of my memory of that time is lost, and if I am reminded then the trauma becomes reawakened. So, I also avoid triggering myself in that way in order to stay well.

Since leaving clinical midwifery practice and moving into academic and research midwifery practice, some have expressed distaste about my having a 'high profile'. So, I can see parallels with the concept of TPS there. A few years ago, an attempt was also made to have me removed from an awards nomination list, after which the award organisers contacted me, concerned for my safety. There have been similar incidents since. So, I really do recognise some of the dysfunctional and deviant behaviours we describe in this chapter. We really need to be lifting each other up instead of tearing one another down.

KM Absolutely. How did all this end?

SP I am not sure if it has. I know the gossip continues more than 10 years on. But I must keep moving forward, learning, growing and thriving to the benefit of the profession.

KM Yes, of course. What helped you get through that experience or is still helping you get through? Were there people, other midwives, who supported you or challenged the deviant behaviour?

SP In my experience, midwives tend to distance themselves from investigations for fear of being blamed themselves. I think if we moved towards compassionate approaches, this would change. In a culture of learning (rather than blame), we can all thrive.

Also, the biggest thing that helped me through the whole event was being fortunate enough to have an independent barrister, who was also a qualified midwife, really fight for me at a time when I just felt hopeless.

KM   Having that person in your corner must have been a big support at the time. Given what you went through and the stress it put you through, it would be understandable if you wanted to call out the people who made that time more difficult than it needed to be.

SP   For the very reasons outlined in this chapter, I have chosen not to name and shame the people who I felt engaged in uncivil behaviour towards me. However, it is important to point out that many registered midwives may not realise that when they 'gossip' or speculate about colleagues' personal circumstances, including health, they may actually be breaching the fundamental tenets of the profession in relation to confidentiality. Ultimately, incivility should be addressed because it can have a serious effect on workplace cultures, and therefore the safety of people receiving care.

KM   That is a really important point. I am sure midwives would never dream of disclosing the health status of someone within their care as it would be considered gross misconduct and have possible legal ramifications, but your experience shows the same standards have not always been applied to colleagues.

SP   Despite my experience happening many years ago now, I still see the same incivility occurring in practice today. There is colossal room for growth in compassionate approaches among midwives and it starts within each of us and how we decide to behave in response to our colleagues.

They tried to bury me, but they didn't realise I was a seed.

– Sinéad O'Connor.

Activity – Identifying Boundaries and Scripting Responses

Personal boundaries are the limits we place around ourselves to ensure our well-being and emotional comfort are maintained. These boundaries are different for all of us, and things we may feel comfortable with, others may not and vice versa. When our boundaries are violated, at work or anywhere else, it can increase levels of stress and strain, and boundaries are more likely to be violated if we don't effectively communicate and assert what they are.

Boundaries are situated around the behaviours we are willing to accept, or not, in others and are related to the emotional response they evoke in us. They may come in the form of physical boundaries (touch, personal space), verbal (the way in which we are spoken to and the words/tone we are willing to accept from others), material (the use and protection of our possessions), or time (how we use and protect our time). The first step to effectively communicating our boundaries at work (or anywhere else) is to have a strong awareness of what they are and how any violation of that boundary affects you emotionally. However, it is important to reflect on your own emotions alongside those of others as asserting your boundary may negatively impact on your relationships with others if approached aggressively or insensitively (the section in Chapter 2 on self-awareness highlights the importance of self and other insights). The key is to be assertive and unambiguous, rather than aggressive or vague. The following activity focuses on boundaries at work but the same steps would work in other areas of your life too.

Step 1: Reflect on your thoughts and emotions around work and people at work. Are there things you are asked to do that make you feel uncomfortable? Does the way someone speaks to you cause negative thoughts or emotions about yourself? Are there any activities, behaviours or expectations around the way that you work that cause emotional discomfort? For example, when my boss calls me on my days off to talk about work issues that are not urgent it means I can't relax on my days off and causes me to feel stressed and worried about work when I should be recovering. Use the space below to make a note of anything that arises for you.

_____

_____

_____

_____

_____

_____

_____

_____

_____

Step 2: Identify what you would like to be different. What behaviours would you like to see instead? What expectations do you have about how you work or how you wish others to work with you? Use the space below to jot down your thoughts.

_____

_____

_____

_____

_____

_____

_____

_____

_____

_____

(*continued*)

(*continued*)

Step 3: Script some clear and assertive statements to use when you feel your boundary may be breached. Include a statement of the behaviour you want to change and why and follow that with a consequence should the undesired behaviour continue. Focus on the behaviour and use 'I' statements (I think... I feel... I would like..., etc.). Offering alternatives gives clarity over what you would like to happen next and these can be framed in a collaborative way ('rather than doing x, could we try doing y'). An example could be, 'This conversation is making me feel uncomfortable due to the language being used and I would like you to use more respectful language. If the tone of the conversation doesn't change, I will leave and we can continue at another time'. Use the space below to write out some statements based on your thoughts in steps 1 and 2.

_____

_____

_____

_____

_____

_____

_____

_____

_____

Step 4: Practise saying your assertive statements out loud. The more you practise, the more natural it will feel if and when you ever need to use them.

CHAPTER 6

Surviving When Things Go Wrong

INTRO TO CHAPTER

Generally, as midwives, we expect to be caring for people going through the physiological process of childbearing. The reason I (Sally) never wanted to be a nurse was because I wasn't keen to provide care to the sick, I was keen to provide care to people who are childbearing. In the context of their role, nurses, along with other healthcare professionals may well go to work every day expecting to experience sickness, death and dying in their work. As such, they may be more prepared to witness such things, whereas midwives, who expected to care for a generally healthy population through a physiological process, may not. It is this proposed deficit in preparedness which may leave midwives more vulnerable to trauma when things go wrong, as ultimately such episodes may be less anticipated in midwifery work.

Nevertheless, things do go wrong in perinatal services and midwives (where trained appropriately) are highly skilled in dealing with obstetric emergencies. Yet it is not always an 'obstetric emergency' when things go wrong. Our professional experiences are far more complex than that. Consequently, in this chapter, we will explore the ways in which things might go wrong in practice and offer solutions as to how you can survive when they inevitably do.

As outlined in Chapter 4, you will notice that there is no mention of 'resilience' in this book as a skill required for survival. This is largely because the term 'resilience' has for some time essentially been used as a stick to beat healthcare staff with through an expectation that the onus is on them to bounce back, or be strong enough to withstand the pressure, rather than on the need for the healthcare workplaces to be safe for staff (e.g. see Gerada 2021). Also, whilst it is true that many traumatising events may be

Surviving and Thriving in Midwifery, First Edition. Sally Pezaro and Karen Maher.
© 2025 John Wiley & Sons Ltd. Published 2025 by John Wiley & Sons Ltd.

unexpected and out of everyone's control (e.g. sudden foetal death with no warning signs), as you will see, there will also be many which nobody should need resilience against (e.g. bullying).

SURVIVING TRAUMATIC INCIDENTS

In relation to surviving 'traumatic incidents', we solicited input from the highly regarded Dr. Jan Smith, a chartered psychologist and the Founder of Healthy You Ltd & MindYourself. The following section is written by Dr. Jan who draws from a wealth of professional experience in nurturing staff. Whilst reading, it is important to note that any event being labelled as 'traumatic' is subjective. In other words, what one person deems to be a traumatic experience, another person may not and vice versa. Equally, the impact of such trauma will vary from person to person. One cannot assume that any single person will be impacted more deeply than another. Though in healthcare, some will be at greater risk than others (e.g. see d'Ettorre et al. 2021).

'It is unlikely that when you entered the midwifery profession, you had to consider how you would "survive" a traumatic workplace incident. Whether you're reading this, having experienced one or not, knowing what trauma might look like in yourself and your colleagues will help prepare you should you ever be in this position. Understanding how you cope when the job you love wounds you not only will support your recovery but also help you stay in your role and thrive in it.

There are different ways that you might be impacted by trauma while at work, known as primary, secondary or vicarious trauma. It is not necessary to get caught up in the definition of these; however, being aware of their symptoms might be helpful, as also the situations that might leave you vulnerable to experiencing them.

Primary and Secondary Trauma

Some examples of work-related situations that can result in direct trauma include being involved in care that has not gone as expected, bullying incidents or experiencing workplace assault. Direct trauma is often the result of an intense event where our physical safety is threatened. Although we might have been involved in situations where we could have experienced trauma, it does not necessarily mean that we will go on to develop trauma-related symptoms.

One key difference between primary and secondary trauma is that we are not in direct danger with the latter. Instead, there is an indirect cause through reading, listening or witnessing a traumatic event. Therefore, we could see a challenging birth with a poor outcome, support a colleague who has suffered a traumatic experience and share their experience and its impact. This could perhaps be your role as their manager, leader or Professional Midwifery Advocate (PMA).

Vicarious Trauma

When we hear, witness or read about multiple traumatic experiences from others, it impacts us. Probably, you might not be able to recall each one; however, they potentially will have an impact. Vicarious trauma accumulates multiple secondary traumatic experiences and is often described as emotional wounding by a thousand stories.

Symptoms of Trauma

Trauma symptoms are on a continuum, with milder symptoms on one end, which intensify as they progress towards the other end to post-traumatic stress disorder (PTSD). Irrespective of where your symptoms might fall on this continuum, all are valid. Our feelings indicate that an event or situation emotionally impacts us. Therefore, we might be more likely to dismiss milder symptoms and carry on thinking they will pass. However, by addressing these, we can prevent their development and support ourselves better. There are crossovers between some of the symptoms and key distinguishable features between direct (primary trauma) and indirect (secondary and vicarious trauma). Additionally, universal symptoms such as sleep disturbances can result from direct and indirect trauma. Figure 6.1 summarises the key symptoms of primary, secondary and vicarious trauma.

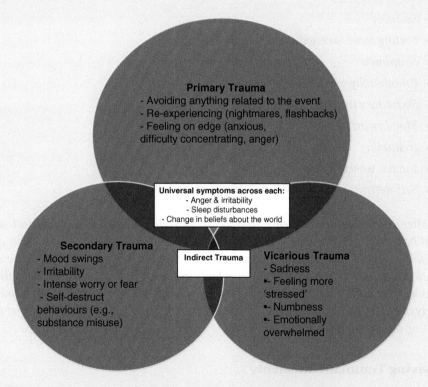

FIGURE 6.1 Key symptoms of primary, secondary and vicarious trauma.

(continued)

(continued)

Trauma and Triggers

Most people recover from a traumatic event. When we have had a traumatic experience, we are likely to be triggered by certain people, places or situations. Being triggered isn't solely about our emotional response. When we experience trauma, our body is flooded with adrenaline. The memory of the event is embedded into our amygdala (a part of our brain responsible for processing fearful and threatening stimuli). It doesn't store the trauma memory like a story; instead, it is processed on a sensory basis. Therefore, the memories of the event are stored through tastes, smells, sounds, touch and visual images.

Primary Trauma

- *Avoiding anything related to the event*
- *Re-experiencing (nightmares, flashbacks)*
- *Feeling on edge (anxious, difficulty concentrating, anger)*

Vicarious Trauma

- *Sadness*
- *Feeling more 'stressed'*
- *Numbness*
- *Emotionally overwhelmed*
- *Secondary trauma*
- *Mood swings*
- *Irritability*
- *Intense worry or fear*
- *Self-destruct behaviours (e.g. substance misuse)*

After a traumatic experience, our brain is trying to understand it, and so it might be that we feel some of the symptoms mentioned in Figure 6.1. Our brain does everything to protect us and keep us safe. However, after trauma, it can perceive safe situations as threatening and prepare our body to respond accordingly, so adrenalin is released. Our flight/fright/freeze/flop response is triggered. Recovering from trauma is largely about helping our brain differentiate between perceived and actual danger and soothing our mind and body.

Surviving Traumatic Incidents

Trying to do as much as we can to support our mind and body calm is undoubtedly helpful, whether you have been impacted by trauma or not. Working in maternity can be emotionally and physically challenging, so finding ways to navigate the potential effect will benefit you. The onus is not exclusively on you to 'survive' a traumatic event. There is a collective responsibility within your team and organisation to create working environments that are trauma-informed and psychologically safe to prevent trauma manifesting after incidents. I have written more extensively about these in two of my books, "Nurturing Maternity Staff: How to tackle trauma, stress and burnout to create a positive working culture in the NHS" and "Managing PTSD for Health and Social Care Professionals: Help for the Helpers". Below are some ways for individuals to manage trauma-related symptoms. Like anything, we want to work optimally; it is key to practice it daily.

Vagus Nerve

During stressful situations, the sympathetic nervous system drives the flight/fright/freeze/flop response, whereas the "rest and digest" state resides in the parasympathetic nervous system. Our vagus nerve is a significant part of this "rest and digest" system and is responsible for our mind-body connection. Therefore, the more toned the vagus nerve is, the more it can support us when needed.

- *Smiling and laughing are simple yet effective ways to activate and tone our vagus nerve.*
- *Humming, singing, chanting and gargling all activate our vagus nerve.*
- *Belly breathing: breathe in slowly, deeply from your belly, and exhale for longer than you inhaled.*

Positive Self-talk

We all have an internal dialogue, and it is sometimes less helpful. When we are under stress or have experienced trauma, thoughts can be more critical and focused on our fears, worsening how we feel. Positive self-talk can support us to reframe the way we think and help us begin to feel more confident. Examples of some statements are:

- *This might be challenging, and I can do this*
- *Right here, right now, I am safe*
- *I have the power to change my mind*
- *I am capable and strong, and I can get through this*
- *Try creating your statements to support you.*

Boundaries

Having boundaries can immensely support our mental health and well-being (see Chapter 5). Often after we've experienced a traumatic incident, it is common for people to feel that life is unpredictable and sometimes unsafe. Boundaries can act to help us feel contained, creating a sense of safety when we are in and away from work. Examples of these might be:

- *I would love to be able to help, but I'm not in a position to, perhaps another time.*
- *I can respect that we have different opinions on this.*
- *I don't feel able to talk about that right now; it isn't the right time.*

(continued)

Reaching Out and Reaching in for Support

When we have been emotionally wounded, reaching out to ask for help might feel overwhelming, particularly when we don't know what we need. The first step could be to share how you feel with someone you trust who is supportive and caring. There are lots of people and organisations who can support you to navigate how you feel, and your GP is also able to help.

When we begin working in maternity, we become part of a community and are responsible for caring for those within it. Checking in on colleagues, asking them "how are you?" and making time for the answer is part of the collective nurturing we should provide to one another. By asking this, it does not mean we take on their struggles or have to have all of the answers because listening to another can be validating and lifesaving. We can all contribute to helping ourselves and our colleagues strive and thrive in maternity'.

Dr. Jan Smith, Chartered Psychologist, Founder of Healthy You Ltd & MindYourself

DEVELOPING PERSONAL INSIGHT AND FORGIVENESS

When things go wrong, the fundamental attribution error trap means we are likely to prefer evidence which supports our existing beliefs rather than alternatives, downplay our personal responsibilities, place undue blame on contextual or external factors and yet reverse all of this when evaluating the failures of others. When we fear the loss of our professional registration and fitness to practise, we can also be tempted to engage in dishonesty, deflection or a 'cover-up' to protect ourselves. Not only is this approach unethical, but it also becomes problematic when we are trying to survive and thrive when things go wrong, ultimately because we simply cannot move forward and thrive following adverse events or transgressions without personal insight and forgiveness. In this section, we will outline how openness and engagement can lead to more favourable outcomes.

In the early stages, midwives and nurses might place blame on external factors and colleagues rather than taking accountability for their own actions. They can also be resentful towards others as they feel pushed to the breaking point (Jones-Berry 2016). Whilst there are indeed many external factors which have undoubtedly contributed to any event taking place in healthcare services, it is the lack of *personal* insight which may stop midwives and nurses from moving forward. A lack of insight following an incident can also result in harsher regulatory sanctions (Gallagher et al. 2022). The activities towards the end of this chapter will also serve to support you in developing personal insight when things go wrong so that you can survive and thrive in moving forward.

As well as the development of insight and remediation when things go wrong, the importance of forgiveness when things go wrong has also been well established (Davis et al. 2015; Ermer and Proulx 2016; Gismero-González et al. 2020). Enright and Fitzgibbons (2000) define forgiveness as the choice to wilfully abandon resentment and related responses, and instead respond to the offender through compassion, unconditional worth, generosity and moral love. Informed by Enright and colleagues' model (Enright and Fitzgibbons 2015), Smallen (2019) proposes a shortened six staged forgiveness practice designed to enable the forgiving of minor transgressions on a routine basis. Thus, in engaging this model regularly, you may in turn have your own abilities strengthened to forgive in the face of more challenging injuries and injustices in future.

Stage One: Identifying Injustice and One's Right to Resentment

- Following the transgression, work towards the acknowledgement that you have been harmed and have a right to feel the way you do.
- Confirm that your interest in forgiving is not a means to gain a sense of moral superiority or to excuse or condone the transgression.
- Once you can confirm that your forgiveness will be sincere and driven by free will, continue to Stage II.

Stage Two: Uncovering with Self-Compassion

- Gently confront any uncomfortable feelings and thoughts associated with the transgression.
- Exercise a caring, non-judgemental and positive regard towards any suffering associated with the transgression.
- Sit with any psychological and physiological discomfort that arises in recalling a transgression long enough to decide to forgive and to extend compassion to a wrongdoer.

Stage Three: Decision to Forgive

- Make a wilful choice to let go of the resentment or anger.
- Offer compassion, benevolence or love towards the offender.
- Say to yourself 'I choose to do no harm'. (e.g. to yourself, other people and/or the perpetrator).
- Sit with this statement and again practise self-compassion where any uncomfortable emotions arise.
- Once you can stand by your decision to 'do no harm', say to yourself 'I choose to forgive'.
- If you can forgive, move to the next stage. If you feel unable to forgive. That's fine. Go straight to stage six.

Stage Four: Reframing and Broadening One's Perspective of the Wrongdoer

- Though it may be challenging, try to reflect upon times when you have done the same or similar action by which you were harmed, allowing empathy to grow.
- As you reflect on your own past actions, repeat the following to yourself 'Just like me. Just like me. Just like me'.
- Try to imagine how the wrongdoer may have been feeling or thinking at the time.

Stage Five: Work and Loving-Kindness

- In softening any feelings of resentment and extending compassion towards the wrongdoer, first speak words to yourself which represent self-compassion such as 'may I be safe, may I be happy, may I be healed'.
- Explore what arises naturally in mind and body in response to these words.
- Repeat similar works of compassion to yourself aimed towards the wrongdoer (e.g. 'may you be safe, may you be happy, may you experience health').

Stage Six: Deepening and Reflection

- Journal reflections upon any new meanings, purpose and awareness that arise from the process.
- Reflect upon what was possible to accomplish and what was difficult.

Though you may wish to continue using this model for regular forgiveness practice, it is important to remember that there is no expectation that there will be a full change of heart towards the wrongdoer early on. Nevertheless, *you will* still gain experience with cultivating compassion in the face of resentment. It is also important to remember that forgiveness should not be a means to gain a sense of moral superiority. Equally, forgiveness does not automatically excuse or condone any transgression.

Looking inwardly, should you find your experiences or behaviours at odds with your professional identity when things go wrong, or your beliefs about surviving trauma at any time, you may equally experience shame defined as 'An intensely painful feeling or experience of believing we are flawed and therefore unworthy of acceptance and belonging' (Brown 2006, p. 45). You may also experience such shame (which can also manifest in withdrawal, avoidance or lashing out) from feeling victimised (Konstam et al. 2001). The problem is that shame does not serve us in any positive way. As discussed in Chapter 5, the shaming of someone else also serves no useful purpose. Shame differs from guilt in that its unhelpful message is that you *are* bad rather than you *did* something bad. If you know you have done something wrong, then you can fix it for next time, right? Whereas shame contrarily allows no room for the remediation needed to move ourselves forward.

Both the development of insight and the process of self-reflection can be uncomfortable. Yet before we can forgive ourselves when things go wrong, we may be arguably worse off trapped in an unproductive cycle of self-condemnation. Woodyatt and Wenzel (2019) usefully propose three potential shifts that need to occur to move from such self-condemnation to self-forgiveness as follows:

1. **Moving from rumination to self-reflection:**
   - Thinking about 'what' is happening on reflection rather than 'why' – is a mindful, non-judging awareness of the situation that allows one to care and act differently in future.
   - Self-distancing through the reconstruction of an experience in generic language (i.e. the generic 'you'), transforming a personal event into a shared universal experience.

- Reflect on the question 'In what way did my actions violate my own values?', then reflect on why that value is important to you, and on times when you act in ways consistent with these values.

2. **Moving from emotions as stressors to emotions as indicators:**
   - Consider that any aversive emotions you feel (e.g. guilt and regret) could be signals of your continued commitment to the values you feel have been violated.

3. **Moving from avoidance to repair:**
   - Sincere expressions of remorse, apologies and forgiveness-seeking can help to restore your moral image, and gain acceptance and forgiveness from others.
   - Taking responsibility for a wrong or harm can reflect your deeper morality, and thus no longer diminish your self-regard.
   - Acting in reducing the risk of repetition can restore values of trust and honesty.
   - Engaging in further repair of self, others and shared relationships can prevent the act from becoming defining of who you are.

Once we can move past any feelings of shame and move into a state where we are ready to forgive (either ourselves or others) we can work on being more insightful in making improvements for the future. It is this insightfulness along with its accompanying remediation which can also serve to reduce the risk of repetition when things have gone wrong. In this sense, we may survive and thrive in coming back stronger when things go wrong. The activity at the end of this chapter will aid you in developing your own personal insight in relation to any future (and past) events.

I can be changed by what happens to me. But I refuse to be reduced by it.
– Maya Angelou

ESCALATING CONCERNS

As experts in physiological pregnancy and childbirth, midwives are in an optimal position to identify when there is cause for concern. At this point, concerns must be escalated to preserve safety. Yet the escalation of concerns can be complex, particularly where midwives feel undervalued and/or are working in unsupportive hierarchies. There is often also some sense of urgency involved, which can in turn exacerbate feelings of stress and therefore psychological well-being and functioning at this time. Emergency protocols should always be observed. Conservative measures may also be taken whilst awaiting conclusive management plans. Yet what else might we consider in the escalation of concerns?

Ultimately, staff must be able to escalate concerns if necessary (Ockenden 2022). Yet in many clinical cases, there can often be a failure to escalate concerns. According to the Royal College of Obstetricians and Gynaecologists (RCOG), the reasons for this largely relate to human factors and behaviour, workload and workforce challenges, and errors in communication methods (Royal College of Obstetricians and Gynaecologists 2020). In challenging these barriers, it will be important to take time (where appropriate) to sit back and reflect on the situation and consider 'what if?' alternatives.

In all cases, it will be important to maintain a 'situational awareness' and an objective overview of a changing situation. In cultivating 'situational awareness', a concept originating from within the aviation industry the following 'NUPA' acronym may be useful (Yoong et al. 2021). Here we have adapted it to reflect a potential scenario in midwifery practice.

N = Notice: 'The more mobile this person is, the more their labour seems to slow'
U = Understand: 'They are probably exhausted and dehydrated'
PA = Project ahead: 'Let's rehydrate and tend to self-care – If the situation continues, we will escalate...'

Equally, we can be challenged in anticipating the loss of situational awareness (e.g. in times of stress) before it occurs. In this task, the minimising of distractions, contingency planning and the continuous evaluation of the 'big picture' will be key. Yet there are warning signs to look for and communicate with others in the identification of reduced situational awareness (Civil Aviation Authority 2016). These include:

- Ambiguity (conflicting information)
- Target fixation (a focus on only one thing)
- Confusion/uncertainty/lack of clarity (often accompanied by psychological distress)
- Failure to pay attention (focused on unimportant activities)
- Failure to meet expected targets
- Failure to adhere to procedures
- Failure to resolve discrepancies (due to conflicting information/personal conflicts)
- Failure to communicate effectively (e.g. vague statements)

When you do escalate, and if colleagues become aggressive, potential escalation can further increase the likelihood of harm. Therefore, the choice of language used to attract attention and level out hierarchical gradients is important. The following CUS and PACE tools may be useful in gaining attention when faced with a steep hierarchical gradient (Green et al. 2017):

I am **(C)**oncerned
I am **(U)**ncomfortable, or this is **(U)**nsafe
I am **(S)**cared–
(P)robe – 'I thought we heard the foetal heartbeat very faintly with some decelerations there?'
(A)lert – 'We need to escalate this to the obstetric team'.
(C)hallenge – 'Please act, I am not happy, this situation needs input from the obstetric team'.
(E)mergency – 'Shout for help. There is no action being taken where there are still concerns in relation to the foetal heartbeat'.

Ultimately, midwives are the experts in physiological pregnancy and childbirth. Yet the communication and escalation of concerns where events fall outside of such boundaries must be done with clarity and confidence. Express what and who you need clearly (e.g. 'obstetric emergency team'). Request for the information to be repeated back to you for clarity. A high-quality handover of information (structured and multidisciplinary) will also be essential in communication and the maintenance of situational awareness overall.

Civility, psychological safety and a supportive culture are key in the escalation of concerns (see Chapter 5). Incivility and hierarchies may have a negative impact upon sound decision-making and result in a reluctance to escalate concerns, increasing risk overall. Strong compassionate and supportive midwifery leadership is required to address culture changes and empower midwives to challenge situations with confidence (see Chapter 8). In this, there must also be clear expectations of accountability, responsibility and the instantiation of strong professional values.

Below is an example of how one midwife, in particular, continues to survive and thrive in escalating concerns, doing so even in the face of adversity:

> *In 2005, I first realised that the recommended routine procedure of immediate clamping had no evidence base, on the contrary, it was causing harm. I thought changing practice would be easy. After all our codes state 'Always practise in line with the best available evidence' …. and immediate cord clamping has none to support it.*
>
> *It has been a long and often difficult journey, but I am still at it. There's still so much work to do before all babies benefit from receiving the full entitlement of their own cord blood as nature intended.*
>
> *I once watched a rugby game and thought of the similarities between changing practice and scoring a rugby try. Running up the field holding onto the ball, ducking and diving and sometimes getting caught at the bottom of a scrum, but you get back up and carry on until you reach your target. It's tough and you get a bit sweaty but just keep going….*
>
> **Amanda Burleigh, RGN, RN, BSc**
> **Midwifery Consultant**

Similarly, the account below is written by a midwife surviving and thriving in India whilst maximising opportunities for learning and escalating concerns for real-world change.

'My name is Inderjeet Kaur, "Indie" to my family, peers and colleagues. I am a British midwife. My career began in the United Kingdom. In 2014, I was invited to visit India to speak on the topic of non-pharmacological pain relief in labour from the midwifery

(continued)

(*continued*)

perspective at the Royal College of Obstetricians and Gynaecologists International Conference in Hyderabad, India. The purpose of my trip also included spending time at the Fernandez Hospital, Hyderabad teaching at their professional midwifery education and training programme. This visit changed my life, indeed, my whole world.

Following my first interaction with Evita, the obstetrician spearheading the midwifery training programme, I volunteered to teach there during my annual leave. I saw that the vision of Fernandez Hospital to promote midwifery in India would face considerable challenges. Evita needed professional support from midwifery colleagues. So, in 2017, I took a sabbatical from my job at the National Health Service, England and went to work as a consultant midwife to train nurses in midwifery at Fernandez Hospital in Hyderabad, India.

In November of that same year, the Government of Telangana, UNICEF and the Fernandez Foundation created the first private/public partnership to train a cohort of 30 nurses as professional midwives. This training changed the landscape of maternal health in Telangana state.

It is essential to know that a nurse trained in India is also certified as a qualified midwife. This is without the additional recommended training of 18 months, which is the global standard set by the International Confederation of Midwives for nurses wanting to be trained as midwives.

The Telangana pilot programme was successful because we had support from qualified midwives at Fernandez and a British midwife, Kate Stringer, who taught at the programme for 12 months. An 18-month curriculum was developed based on the ICM global standards of clinical competencies. The midwifery team led the theory sessions with obstetricians teaching medical complications.

The obstetrical environment and challenges faced during the training made me more determined to persist on this journey. The training occurred in high-volume, public hospitals with a solid medical-led team of obstetricians side-by-side with experienced midwives. Clinical leadership and respectful maternity care were taught and modelled by the trainers as they worked alongside the trainees. We had to be the new role models for the trainees, breaking down their experiences of obstetric violence and building up a deep understanding of the philosophy and practice of midwifery.

In many medically dominated obstetrical environments, pregnancy, labour and birth are not seen as physiological events in a woman's life but as catastrophes waiting to happen. Therefore, care during labour and birth is routinely and inappropriately medicalised.

Midwifery is a sea change in obstetrical care in India. We teach the trainees to help women give birth while standing by the mother's side, in contrast to doctors who stand at the bottom of the bed with women in stirrups. We ensure women are upright and mobile during labour and use gym balls and rebozo to help cope with the pain of childbirth. Finally, women are encouraged to give birth in positions of their choice. Eventually, a big milestone – stirrups were removed from birthing tables.

The vast majority of women in India are birthing alone and experience unnecessary interventions to expedite birth. The pillars of midwifery practice are non-intervention, respect and compassion. This question from an HIV positive labouring woman gives us pause. "Why are you being so kind to me?" she asked. With her first birth, she had experienced severe trauma. She was physically abused and discriminated against. Her care with our midwives made her feel cared for and respected. On reflection, our trainees shared that they were learning to practice respectful women-centred care for "every" woman.

It is a challenge to survive in an environment where we are surrounded by practices such as unnecessary, frequent pelvic exams in labour by multiple providers, routine episiotomies, fundal pressure, immediate cord clamping and separation of the new-born from the mother. And, in contrast to the midwifery model of informed consent, all these interventions are performed without any consent.

Let me illustrate the severity of the problem by sharing this story. While working on the labour and delivery ward, I came upon an obstetrician performing a vaginal examination while talking on her mobile. This was particularly distressing to me because we had just spent time that day educating all staff about the need for informed consent before any invasive exam or procedure such as vaginal exams (VE) and episiotomies. The doctor was performing a VE without the woman's consent. The labouring woman said she did not want the doctor to perform the vaginal examination, however, the obstetrician continued to do so without consent while on her mobile. I was shocked. I felt like I would be colluding with this disrespectful practice if I did nothing. Therefore, I shared my experience with the Telangana Commissioner of Health and Family Welfare, the visionary leader who initiated and strongly supported the midwifery training programme for the State's public hospitals. She is a firm believer in respectful maternity care and responded with swift action. This kind of accountability at the hospital in State and Government of India levels is critical to the transformation of obstetrical care that is so desperately needed throughout India.

Radical changes are occurring. The first batch of 30 qualified midwives, posted in teams of 3 across 10 public health facilities, have turned the tide. Normal [undisturbed physiological] births have increased, C-sections have decreased and women are happier with their birth experience.

The Ministry of Health, Delhi, noticed these changes, leading to India's commitment to establish midwifery-led care units across its public hospitals.

*The training cascaded to obstetric colleagues with whom we shared evidence-based practices that challenged present norms. Open and respectful discussions slowly paved the way for trainees to practise what they had learned. And their practices are evidence that the midwifery model is safe, effective and well accepted by women. The 30 qualified midwives share how they helped save lives in their facilities in cases of postpartum bleeding or severe hypertension with signs of imminent eclampsia. **Post Partum Haemorrhage** (PPH) is the cause of 25% of maternal deaths in India (WHO). These deaths are preventable when midwives have been trained to global professional standards of midwifery practice.*

The evidence is in. Normal [undisturbed physiological] births increased. Midwives dealt effectively with shoulder dystocia, vaginal breech births, severe hypertension, eclampsia and PPH.

(continued)

(continued)

I am humbled to be given the privilege of making a difference in India's quality of maternity services. My belief in midwifery training has been firmly reinforced, and the work here has given a new purpose to my life'.

Inderjeet Kaur
Director of Midwifery Services
Fernandez Foundation, Hyderabad, India

MAXIMISING OPPORTUNITIES FOR LEARNING

When things go wrong, it is essential that we learn from our mistakes and improve our future practices. Whilst failure is difficult to confront for both individuals and organisations, negative outcomes though unsettling, are highly valuable in learning. A useful illustration of this lies in Karl Popper's (1959) black swan thought experiment, where it was hypothesised that all swans were white. Yet in searching for, and constantly finding white swans we reveal nothing about whether all swans *are* white. Consequently, finding a black swan holds far superior informational value, because it allows us to know more. Thus, to maximise opportunities for learning, we must similarly apportion equal energy towards seeking information about what went wrong to that with which we apportion to what went right. Ultimately, incident investigations must be meaningful for families and staff, and lessons must be learned and implemented in practice in a timely manner (Ockenden 2022). Yet how do we go about this?

Edmondson (2011) published several 'Strategies for learning from failure' in the *Harvard Business Review* where it is critical to establish the necessary culture, systems and procedures to learn from failure. Strategies included:

- Building a learning (rather than blaming) culture – ask 'what happened?' – not 'who did it?'
- Detecting failure early and dissecting it
- Encouraging open discussions when things go wrong
- Welcoming questions
- Displaying humility along with curiosity
- Thoroughly analysing failure
- Promoting experimentation

Edmondson ends poignantly with the following quote:

Those that catch, correct, and learn from failure before others do will succeed. Those that wallow in the blame game will not.

Once a failure has been detected, it's essential to go beyond obvious and superficial reasons to understand the root causes thoroughly and appropriately. For example, all post-mortem examinations must be conducted by a pathologist who is an expert in physiology and pregnancy-related pathologies (Ockenden 2022). There are also several systematic tools to assist perinatal teams in learning from failure, each of which has trade-offs (Hagley et al. 2019; Harel et al. 2016). Thus, it is suggested that an amalgamation of tools such as root cause analysis and incident analysis frameworks are combined to ensure coherence. Whilst the selection of tools may vary depending on the context of the healthcare organisation, their use should improve the reliability, safety and quality of care provided in their localities.

Haxby and Shuldham (2018) usefully outline the steps involved in undertaking a root cause analysis:

1. Getting started
2. Gathering and mapping the information
3. Identifying care and service delivery problems
4. Analysing the information
5. Identifying contributory factors and root causes
6. Generating recommendations and solutions
7. Implementing solutions
8. Writing the investigation report
9. Continuing to implement solutions and monitoring progress

In your analyses, it can be useful to use the 'five whys' technique (Serrat 2017), which suitably shifts us away from thinking about who? And into why? An example of using this technique is presented below and adapted from materials developed by the National Patient Safety Agency:

1. The birthing parent deteriorated – why?
2. Because they received the wrong medication – why?
3. Because it was given in error – why?
4. Because the label was misread – why?
5. Because medicines with similar names are stored together – why?
   - Because these medicines are stored alphabetically

Harel et al. (2016) also recommend the following tools in root cause analysis:

- The Fishbone/Ishikawa/cause and effect diagrams resemble a fish skeleton where the problem (effect) is written in a box on the far right and a central 'spine' is drawn to the left of the box in which the problem is recorded. Diagonal 'fish bones' are then drawn coming off the central 'spine'. This visual tool is used to brainstorm about the main causes of a quality-of-care outcomes/problem and the sub-causes leading to each main cause.
- Process mapping (flow charts) can be used to understand all the different steps and improvement opportunities that take place in a complicated system.

- Pareto charts (where data can be observed and collected repeatedly (e.g. through audits and interviews) can equally be used to visualise which causes represent the two or three most common causes of the quality-of-care problem/outcome.

Once you have completed your root cause analyses, the following elements should be included in reporting according to guidelines published by Haxby and Shuldham (2018):

- Incident details – description, date, type (category), effect on patient, severity
- Background and context – information about the organisation, the service or the area in which the incident occurred such as the number of beds, patients and staff, and information about previous similar incidents
- Terms of reference – why the investigation and report is being undertaken, members of the investigation team
- Involvement of the patient and their family in accordance with the duty of candour – whether and how they have been kept informed of the incident and the investigation
- Involvement and support of the staff involved – whether and how the staff involved have been debriefed and offered support
- Information and evidence gathered, including the methodology used for this – how relevant information was collected in the investigation
- How the root cause analysis was undertaken and the tools that were employed
- Identification of the incident – when and how the incident was first identified
- Narrative chronology of events – a straightforward account of what happened in date and time order, written clearly using complete sentences, like an essay
- Timeline – the 'what' information, giving precise dates and times of the significant events written in the form of a table
- Notable practice – the good aspects of the care and service delivery
- Care and service delivery problems identified
- Relevant issues – the relevant contributory factors identified in the investigation
- Lessons learned – areas for change to prevent similar incidents recurring
- Recommendations – corrective actions and changes to practice to make care safer
- Action plan – the SMART (specific, measurable, achievable, realistic and time-bound) actions that will be undertaken, and what is to be done, by whom and when, as well as the measures that will be employed to mitigate risk
- Monitoring – identifying who has the responsibility for overseeing the implementation of the action plan, as well as the audit and data monitoring to measure the effectiveness of the actions taken
- Reporting and sharing – identifying who should receive the report and who will ensure it is distributed to them and by when

Learning from failure is challenging, particularly for those who are typically admired for determination, proficiency and action. Moreover, in examining our own failures we may be simultaneously eroding our self-esteem. Failure carries an irrefutable (yet often unwarranted) stigma, which leads to people staying silent and lessons from failure unlearnt. Still, it is suggested that whilst some reasons for failure are blameworthy (e.g. deviance, inattention and lack of ability), others are praise-worthy (e.g. hypothesis testing, uncertainty and exploratory testing) according to Edmondson (2011). Thus, the rewards of learning from failure may only be fully realised in building a culture of psychological safety in which the value of learning from failure can be celebrated. To avoid things going wrong in the first place, we can also embrace the following seven features of safety in perinatal services: (i) commit-ment to safety and improvement at all levels, with everyone involved; (ii) technical competence, supported by formal training and informal learning; (iii) teamwork, cooperation and positive working relationships; (iv) constant reinforcing of safe, eth-ical and respectful behaviours; (v) multiple problem-sensing systems, used as the basis of action; (vi) systems and processes designed for safety, and regularly reviewed and optimised; (vii) effective coordination and ability to mobilise quickly (Liberati et al. 2021). Incorporating new thinking about how safety is created (e.g. via Safety II/resilient healthcare) is also required if we are to continue to improve safety and quality in perinatal services (Anderson and Watt 2020). It will also be important to further explore connections between employee and organisational outcomes and patient outcomes in future, where information is currently lacking (Bernstein et al. 2021).

Further reading on this topic can be found in the recommended resources section at the end of the book.

Ultimately, nobody should be silenced in pursuit of maximising opportunities for learning. When listening, it will be important to develop caring and transparent com-plaints response processes which involve service users (Ockenden 2022). Themes and trends must also be consistently monitored by governance teams.

IN CONVERSATION (KAREN AND SALLY EXPLORE PERSONAL INSIGHT INTO WHAT HAPPENS WHEN THINGS GO WRONG)

KM It can be difficult to talk about when things go wrong. It can trigger some negative emotions, but it would be interesting to learn from your own reflections on times when things haven't gone to plan.

SP I have survived traumatic incidents as a midwife. I have also failed to manage my health at times. For years, I held a lot of shame in relation to what had happened to me both personally and professionally. This was overwhelmingly influenced by others who I felt attempted to shame me in addition to my own sense of shame. Of course, the wonderful Brené Brown assures us that 'if we share our shame story with the wrong person, they can easily become one more piece of flying debris in an already dangerous storm', and for a long time I was indeed convinced that once I shared my story, I would only be shamed further by the wrong people hearing my story. The first time I decided to tell my story years later was as part of the stakeholder group to the study 'Care Under Pressure 2: Caring for the Carers'. I shocked myself at how emotional

I was in retelling my story, even in this safe space. The response was awe-inspiringly compassionate and empathetic as I was telling the 'right people' my story.

KM I think that highlights the power in having that safe space to share what happened. It helps us process and make sense of our experience as well as giving others the opportunity to learn from our experience if that is what is needed. How has it shaped how you respond to when things go wrong for others?

SP I use my own experiences in safe spaces now to help others learn from it and grow. I also aim to be compassionate, kind and fair towards others when things go wrong. I have spent years dedicated to midwifery workforce research too in a bid to ensure that what I went through doesn't happen to others.

I think I have had just about every symptom of primary, secondary and vicarious trauma outlined by Dr. Jan Smith in this chapter. Nevertheless, when you lack insight into your own health and well-being you can't always step back and identify these things at the time. I wish I had the tools and knowledge back then that I have now.

KM I can understand that, however, without that experience, you don't know whether you would have the insight you do today or whether you would be using it to help others on their journey. You have certainly shown how it is possible to turn what was a difficult and negative experience into personal growth and positive actions since that time. With that in mind, what would you like others to know about the process that might help them through the experience?

SP When things go wrong, the thought of investigations can be terrifying. It can feel as if a part of your identity is being scrutinised. Yet it's important to use these incidents as an opportunity to learn and grow.

KM Having others see your potential and the possibility for things to be different can help you see it in yourself.

SP That is true, but it can certainly *feel* like the world is against you. The activity on developing insight presented in this chapter is of my own design following my own experiences.

Ultimately, opening up enabled a swifter recovery for me and allowed me to gain insight and forgive myself much sooner than I would have been able to otherwise.

KM Absolutely, being open about what went wrong allows you to move towards healing. How has that healing been for you?

SP I have learnt that empathy and compassion are the antidote to shame. I worked through my own forgiveness a long time ago. I could never have moved forward and got to where I am now without it. I would have been no use to anyone, let alone the midwifery profession had I continued to live in shame.

KM Thank you for being so open about your experiences. I am sure there are people who may read this and who may find comfort in the fact they are not the only ones going through such a difficult time and will be helped by the tools and advice you have given.

Activity – Working with Insight

According to Price et al. (2021, p. 999), insight relates to 'a readiness to explore others' perceptions of one's own behaviour or performance, and to validate those perceptions; and acceptance that one's own performance or behaviour is divergent from accepted standards'. Such insight is considered essential in personal remediation, which in turn reduces the risk of repetition (e.g. see Prescott-Clements et al. 2017).

If something has gone wrong in relation to your practice, this may invoke negative emotions, such as anger and shame. You may also be fearful of sanctions or judgement. However, it will be important to find a safe space in which to unearth your own personal insight. The development of trusting relationships will also be a key enabler in this process. If you have access to a union or workplace representative, we strongly suggest you engage with them as soon as any investigations begin.

Activity 1: Developing Insight

Reflecting on an incident where something has gone wrong in practice, write a list of everything that has contributed to the problem, anything that passes in your thought process. Second, write another list of everything you personally could or should have done differently in relation to the incident. Make both lists as long as you possibly can. Now, remove the first list entirely. What is left is the start of your own personal insight. It's not that the first list doesn't matter, but rather you are decisively remaining focused on the things you can personally reflect on, acknowledge and remediate.

We have presented a short example of this below. This hypothetical example focuses on an incident relating to conduct. However, you could equally relate it to a personal health-related issue by reflecting on how you could or should have managed your health more appropriately. You can also relate this exercise to a clinical competence issue such as a medication error.

Activity 2: Getting to the Bottom of the Problem

It can be tempting to minimise the problem when things go wrong. Yet the trivialisation of an episode can prevent you from developing true insight and reflection. To help you move past this, let us adapt the 'five whys' technique (Serrat 2017) to ask, '*Why is that a problem?*' in the hypothetical example below:

1. I posted unprofessional pictures of myself in my uniform at work on social media – why is that a problem?
2. Because the public will see a midwife acting unprofessionally at work – why is that a problem?
3. Because the public may lose trust in midwives – why is that a problem?
4. Because if the public lose trust in midwives, they may stop engaging with the profession – why is that a problem?

(continued)

(*continued*)

5. Because those in need of midwifery care may not receive it – why is that a problem?
   - Because an absence of midwifery care may result in increased morbidity and ultimately in some cases, death.

This hypothetical example may seem extreme. Yet it is this level of granularity which allows you to explore the ripple effects of risk associated with a particular episode.

Activity 3: Reducing the Risk of Repetition

Once you have developed personal insight and got to the bottom of the problem, you have a positive and unique opportunity to engage in remediation and thus reduce risks of repetition. In this, it will be important to identify the tangible ways in which you can do this. Let's make a list of hypothetical examples from which you can draw and add to (see Tables 6.1 and 6.2).

These lists provided in relation to possible remedial actions to hypothetical situations are not exhaustive. In making your own lists, it will be important to list and action as many remedial actions as possible. In this task, you will need to ensure that all remedial actions directly address the issues raised (e.g. training in relation to record keeping when an issue related to record keeping is identified).

TABLE 6.1   Example of insight following hypothetical critical incident.

Contextual issues	Personal insight
I have seen many colleagues do the same thing and they have never gotten in trouble about this before – I am being victimised!	Whilst other people may do this, it was still unacceptable according to the professional standards expected of me.
I was never told not to do this.	I should have taken responsibility for finding out what my professional responsibilities were in this case. I was in a position of authority at the time.
Nobody was harmed by what I did	It was fortunate that nobody was harmed by what I did. However, I did put people at risk of harm.
I asked my friends and they said they would do the same thing in my situation	Whilst my friends are trying to make me feel better, they are not a registered midwife like myself. I need to take responsibility for my own actions as a registered midwife.
The systems in place let me get away with this. They should have been fixed if they didn't want me to do it.	The systems were indeed broken. However, I took advantage of that fact by taking shortcuts rather than highlighting the potential for concern.

TABLE 6.2 Example of potential actions following insight.

Problem in need of remediation	Possible remedial actions
Health: I am drunk on shift. I am impaired by reason of my alcohol addiction.	• Remove yourself from the workplace and communicate the need for your absence. • Seek professional help and engage fully in prescribed programmes of recovery. • Write a reflective statement. • Seek medical reports to document progress.
Competence: I made various medicines management and record keeping errors.	• Request supervision. • Undertake further (preferably assessed) training related to medicines management and record keeping errors. • Write a reflective statement. • Maintain training certificates.
Conduct: I breached professional boundaries when supporting a client through pregnancy. I also viewed the medical records of their partner unnecessarily.	• End any residual inappropriate relationships in a professional manner. • Write a reflective statement. • Undertake further (preferably assessed) training related to topics such as the maintenance of professional boundaries, confidentiality, information governance and professionalism.

CHAPTER 7

Thriving in Evidence-based Practice and Academia

INTRO TO CHAPTER

As we have mentioned before, midwives don't just catch babies, and so it is important to explore how one might contribute to the wider roles in midwifery (See Chapter 2). Nevertheless, in all roles, it will be vital in every aspect of your professional midwifery journey to remain an evidence-based practitioner. This essentially means immersing yourself in both 'research' and 'education' as a life-long learner. In combining these two concepts, theories around 'research inspired teaching' (RIT) in midwifery have long fascinated me (Sally), and so led me to co-create with those who purported to engage in it. From this work, we were able to co-create definitions of both teaching, research and RIT as follows.

Teaching involves 'an intellectual partnership between the educator and the self-actuated learner, where both are engaged in co-creating, understanding, critiquing and applying knowledge to particular contexts, thereby developing new transferable skills and understandings together'.

Co-creators defined research as:

a process of inquiry which draws insights from different perspectives and practices and leads on to the creation of new knowledge or the use of existing work in new and creative ways to generate new understandings through critical analysis to inspire, instigate positive societal changes and inform both practice and innovation.

Surviving and Thriving in Midwifery, First Edition. Sally Pezaro and Karen Maher.
© 2025 John Wiley & Sons Ltd. Published 2025 by John Wiley & Sons Ltd.

Co-creators decided that RIT is:

> *Where research is embedded throughout all teaching, learning and assessment activities and content as part of an authentic, disruptive and evidenced-based exploration, in which both self-actuated learners and educators are committed and inspired toward critical thinking and the co-creation of innovative new knowledge, understandings, transferable skills and 'real world' impact together. (Pezaro et al. 2022a)*

Keep these definitions in mind throughout this chapter, where we hope to inspire you and enable you to thrive in both evidence-based practice and academia. The importance of evidence-based practice and academia in midwifery cannot be underestimated. Yet it can take up to 17 years for research evidence to have a direct impact upon healthcare (Morris et al. 2011). Implementation science in midwifery may be one way to speed up the process. For a practical guide on how to use some of the innovative approaches to identifying, understanding and overcoming barriers to the adoption, adaption, integration, scale-up and sustainability of evidence-based interventions used by implementation scientists, see the example of midwifery-led continuity of care (MLCC) as an illustration see Harris et al. (2019). We can also ensure that we remain evidence-based practitioners throughout our professional midwifery journeys by immersing ourselves in the literature and keeping abreast of any new research which comes available to us.

We hope that this chapter may also assist in the bridging of this gap somewhat by demonstrating the various ways in which research and evidence can be brought together and applied in practice, and how midwives themselves can be galvanised into pursuing midwifery careers in both research and education.

The state of the world's midwifery report (Nove et al. 2021) advocates the need for attention towards the theory– practice balance and transformative education, promoting research and academic activities at every level. Still, I (Sally) personally struggled through school and early academia, and I remember battling with the same things I try to mentor others through now. The following chapter is the one I wish I'd had as a budding academic midwife. I hope it brings you the same 'light-bulb' moments.

TYPICAL EXPECTATIONS AND TIPS FOR CAREER ADVANCEMENT

We both (Sally and Karen) work in academia. We both have had non-traditional routes to becoming academics, having spent the early parts of our careers in practice and coming back to study later in life. Psychology arguably has stronger roots in academia, with many psychologists holding doctorates and climbing the academic ladder, so there is a well-trodden career path in academia for psychologists. However, we observe far fewer midwives with PhDs or in leadership posts within higher education. Academic midwifery is not always valued highly, hence the state of the world's midwifery report's call for midwifery leadership in these areas.

Future generations of midwives will always need to be taught, upskilled and nurtured. Therefore, there will always be a need for midwifery educators both in practice and within higher education institutions. Yet it is important to consider how such educators may maintain their authority to teach by staying ahead of the game. If you become a midwifery educator, the four types of scholarship, as originally put forth by Boyer (1990) may enable you to do this:

Discovery: generation of new knowledge and sharing that knowledge with our community (e.g. primary research shared at conferences or disseminated through publication).

Integration: taking knowledge and synthesising it into something that is useful for practice (e.g. a case study with a literature review published or shared at a conference)

Application: putting knowledge into practice (e.g. serving in committees or contributing to guidelines)

Teaching: development of educational programmes or resources (e.g. presenting to faculty members, students and peers with authority on a topic of interest).

Whilst some institutions may either be more teaching or research focused, it will be important to think about how your own academic practice may have an influence upon both throughout your career. To enhance your teaching, seek out opportunities for academic development in pedagogical practice (e.g. Postgraduate Certificate in Academic Practice in Higher Education [*PgCAPHE*]). To enhance your practice in research, seek out smaller method based educational opportunities, or a research degree such as a master's in research or a Doctor of Philosophy (PhD), which will prepare you to think like a researcher and approach problem-solving in new and diverse ways. You may be able to get a PhD funded by your institution as part of their investment in you. You can also search for studentship opportunities offered around the world (e.g. via www.findaphd.com).

Attend as many conferences and learning opportunities as you can. Watch how others thrive in academia and seek out what works best for you. Get to know the key works in your field of midwifery expertise. Who is publishing where? Who is writing what? Academia and evidence-based practice are constantly evolving. Stay on top of the conversation and see how you might contribute in meaningful ways. Seek out problems to solve and new impactful avenues to explore. A strong contribution in research and academia can change the world.

Not everyone wins a scholarship or a fellowship. Academia is challenging and involves a lot of rejection. There is no single explanation for how you might expect your career to advance in academic midwifery, and timings may also depend on what your academic goals are. Whilst many academics may be successful in becoming professors before they turn 40 years old, midwives (as with other health professionals) may bring a wealth of clinical experience with them prior to academia. This may mean that this is something you come to later in your career, though not necessarily.

In the excerpt below, Fiona Gibb, Director of Professional Midwifery at the Royal College of Midwives and Associate Lecturer at Robert Gordon University offers some insights on a midwifery career in research and academia along with advice to support other midwives looking to thrive in this area.

'My journey as a qualified midwife in academia began in 2007 and working in the NHS, I regularly supported and assessed student midwives, which sparked my interest in education career pathway. I volunteered to take part in support facilitation of learning events in the hospital and consequently completed formal clinical instructor training with NHS Education for Scotland to teach resuscitation and exam of the newborn courses. Being active in practice education provided the link to the local university and I became an associate lecturer teaching midwifery theory and clinical skills. This was my first step into academia and the experience proved valuable to gaining a lecturer post two years later.

An unseen aspect of being an academic is often the requirement to return to formal study as a student and a postgraduate teaching qualification was excellent support during the early years and was recognition of the day-to-day work. Later, a research study exploring service user involvement in midwifery education was awarded a master's degree in research which supported a promotion to senior lecturer and Lead Midwife for education in 2017. To deliver high-quality education involves the continued awareness of evidence-based practice and research. The balance of a busy workload and continuing your own professional development is an ongoing challenge but choosing the right courses and being able to use your experiences towards formal qualification helped to stay on track.

There have been numerous challenges along the way: developing a new curriculum to implement the Future Midwife standards for education, line management and leadership development, not to mention redesigning a course in response to a global pandemic. Support from others, internally and externally to source collective wisdom and consensus proved most useful in challenging times. Establishing collaborative networks is essential for prompt decision-making and support for each other and for students, as well as celebrating achievements. Collaboration can prove a hurdle as universities work in a competitive environment, however, a shared commitment to excellent education and maternity care provides motivation and encourages progress. I continue to embrace the challenges and mistakes and have not stopped learning. Here is what I've learnt so far:

If considering an academic career pathway, actively seek out opportunities to be involved in the facilitation of education whether that be working with students or practice education teams. Become known for an interest in education and research which will support further opportunities to work their way back to you.

It can be a struggle to get back into study after time away from it. Target professional development that supports your goal. Speak with those already working with roles that you aspire to or look at the person specification requirements for those roles and consider what your development needs are and prioritise them first.

Be prepared to continue to learn and manage competing demands. Consider how your day-to-day work can contribute towards a qualification, rather than view as an additional demand on time. For example, a quality improvement project can contribute to a teaching qualification or a research study.

Collaborative networks and a shared sense of purpose can help through the best and most challenging of times. Seek out others who may help your journey or learn *from others how they have addressed similar challenges. This may be through pre-existing national groups, or informally through events and social media.'*

Fiona Gibb
MRes, PgCert HELT, BM, RM, SFHEA
Director of Professional Midwifery, Royal College of Midwives
Associate Lecturer, Robert Gordon University

TOP 10 TIPS FOR ACADEMIC SUCCESS

As academics used to marking both student essays and reviewing academic papers prior to publication we are well versed in seeing the same mistakes happen over and over again. So, in this short section, we aim to highlight 10 broad tips for academic success so that you may avoid making some of the same mistakes we see in academic practice.

1. All healthcare professionals will need to write about their 'practice' a lot. Yet so often 'practic(s)e' is spelled incorrectly and/or interchangeably within a document. The verb 'to practise' is spelled with an 's', yet the noun where practice is a *thing* is spelled with a 'c'. If you are not sure about this when writing, then try to use the word *advice* or *advise* in the sentence. Whichever sounds correct informs you as to whether you should spell practice with either a 'c' or an 's' in that context. *Note – this is not the case for American English spellings!*

2. Appendices go after the reference lists. So often we see appendices come before the reference list. This weakens the structure of the document.

3. Always refer to appendices, tables and figures in the main text... (e.g. "the demographics of all participants are presented in table 1").

4. Avoid making bold statements of fact without citation to evidence. This remains the case, even if something is common knowledge such as 'smoking causes lung cancer'.

5. Be careful when citing non-academic literature to support your arguments. For example, a nursing magazine may well have an article claiming new facts and figures which support your point. However, the nursing magazine will likely be quoting from a peer reviewed piece of evidence. It is this original source you need to find, make your own interpretation of their work, and then cite. The same is true for those using dictionaries to cite definitions – avoid this and stick to citing peer reviewed articles.

6. Avoid large chunks of text that dilute your arguments. Shorter paragraphs which hold one argument per paragraph strengthen the structure of your work. Subheadings may help you in breaking up large sections of text also.

7. Avoid overly long sentences. The structure of your work will be much improved if you can keep sentences short and to the point. Aim for one concept linked to a maximum of one other for each sentence.

8. Take inspiration from other academic work published in the literature. One can gain significant inspiration from the writing style of others and the structure upon which other peer reviewed articles are based, so lots of reading can help your own writing. For example, you may find that the presentation of results in one academic article simplifies complex information in a particularly useful way. In this sense, you may choose to present the results you expect to get in the same format to gain the same benefits. However, it is important to avoid plagiarism (misrepresenting someone else's work as your own) so never cut and paste from other people's work. The aim is to interpret and integrate your reading of others' work into your own personal informed line of argument.

9. Start writing drafts early so that you can keep coming back to your work with fresh eyes each time. A last-minute job may result in a compromise on quality and potential mistakes in citations, risking plagiarism.

10. Be minimal in description and maximum on critical analysis and evaluation. Try to round off every paragraph with a concluding argument. At the end of every paragraph ask yourself... So what? What does this mean? What am I saying?

Indeed, critical thinking and critical analysis are crucial in midwifery work. We do it every day in clinical practice, but how might we do the same in academia? Whilst still important, we need to go beyond description to make sense of the concepts we are dealing with, draw from the wider literature and ultimately make evidence-based arguments and conclusions to demonstrate evaluation, critical thinking and analysis.

The following is an example taken from one of my (Sally's) published academic articles (Pezaro et al. 2022a). We will use a paragraph from this work to demonstrate the different elements of description, analysis drawing from the wider literature and evaluation. When these three elements come together, critical analysis is achieved.

'The very real prospect of criminal sanctions for those midwives who divert medications from whom they were intended in the workplace can be complex to navigate (Pezaro et al. 2022a). **Some courts are divided on whether an individual with an addiction who commits an unlawful act is beyond the reach of criminal law because the act is then considered to be involuntary (Sidhu 2020). Yet ultimately, there is a need to pursue individualised approaches to investigations.** Thus, before engaging law enforcement, employers and policy makers may usefully decipher between acts against probity (e.g. intent to supply) and behavioural symptoms of ill health, such as those presented in this sample (Pezaro et al. 2021a). Equally, the unnecessary involvement of law enforcement may be avoided by ensuring that there is congruence between policies which relate to theft/dishonesty and policies which relate to drug, alcohol and substance use.'

- *Description*
- ***Analysis drawing from the wider literature***
- Evaluation

Can you pull out the same elements in other academic articles or your own work? Can you improve on the paragraph above? Each element comes together to make a whole argument or conclusion. The elements together complete the task, yet so often we find that only the first two are present.

Table 7.1 may offer further insights into the types of questions you may ask yourself to ensure that every academic argument involves a comprehensive description, analysis and evaluation in demonstrating critical thinking and analysis.

TABLE 7.1   Critical thinking questions.

Description: an introductory background to contextualise the topic	What?	What is this about?
		What is the context/background here?
		What is the problem to be explored?
	Where?	Where does it take place? (e.g. local, national, international clinical setting, geopolitical space?)
	Who?	Who may be affected?
		Who does this involve?
		Who might care about this?
	When?	Time? date?
		A particular period in childbearing (e.g. antenatal)?
Analysis: engaging with the wider literature exploring possibilities and the different parts in relation to both one another and everything all together	How?	How did this occur?
		How does it work?
		How is the methodology used to answer the question?
		How is the theory engaged here?
		How does one thing affect another?
		How does everything fit together as a whole?
	Why?	Why is this important?
		Why was this done?
		Why not something else?
		Why did this happen?
	What if?	What if this is wrong?
		What are the alternatives?
		What if something else was removed or added?
Evaluation: conclusions and recommendations for future action and research, along with potential solutions and implications	So what?	What is significant about this?
		What does this mean?
		What is convincing about this?
		What are the implications?
	What next?	What are the possibilities?
		Where else might this be applicable?
		What are the lessons learnt?
		What now?
		What next?

WRITING FOR PUBLICATION

So, you may ask yourself, why as a midwife you would want to write for publication. Well first of all, we know from experience that there are many amazing midwifery initiatives and research projects being conducted around the world and if you are doing something good, it is worth sharing with others. Equally, if you are doing a midwifery project, a publication acts as a project output and a record of what has taken place. You may also use a publication to support further applications for funding or to evidence research excellence. Put simply, an accurate publication is essentially recorded 'verification' of what happened. A blind peer review of your work can also give your work further credibility in status. You as a midwife may also achieve increased status in your field by having your work published, and consequentially, you will have increased subject authority in your area.

There are different types of publications in which you may choose to share your work. Each of these will have a different purpose and structure.

Editorial: Where you simply have a pertinent comment to make, an idea to share or news to disseminate. These are generally quite short and dependent upon what the journal is willing to publish.

- Example: Pezaro, S., Maher, K., and Fissell, M. (2022). Midwives need a useable past to shape their future. The Lancet 399 (10329): 1046–1047.

Research article: These articles will usually share original research studies reviewed by expert 'peers' in the field prior to publication. Word counts again depend on journal submission requirements.

- Example: Pezaro, S., Maher, K., Bailey, E. and Pearce, G. (2022). Problematic substance use in midwives registered with the United Kingdom's Nursing and Midwifery Council: a pragmatic mixed methods study. Midwifery: 103409.

Discussion/position piece: Usually slightly longer than an editorial, these articles may draw more widely from the literature and present more theory driven approaches in relation to interesting debates, discussions and ideas.

- Example: Pezaro, S. and Maher, K. (2021). Midwives' substance use. British Journal of Midwifery 29 (4): 190–191.

Book/Chapter: Books and book chapters may be used to convey a compendium of your work in a more conversational manner to more specific audiences. You may have more autonomy and authority over the way in which these are structured and presented.

- Example: The book you are reading right now...

Monograph: In some fields, monographs are used as a detailed written study of a single specialised subject or an aspect of it

- Example: Bradley, M., Leonard, V., and Totelin, L. (2021). *Bodily Fluids in Antiquity*. Abingdon: Routledge, p. 452.

Review: A review article will report on a particular type of review of the literature which has been conducted, of which there are many.

- Example: Pezaro, S., Patterson, J., Moncrieff, G., and Ghai, I. (2020). A systematic integrative review of the literature on midwives and student midwives engaged in problematic substance use. Midwifery, 102785.

Case Study: This type of article will typically be a report on one intensive exploration conducted on one particular person, intervention, or group.

- Example: Thorpe, D., Neiman, S., White, J., and Pezaro, S. (2022). A Midwifery team's journey through implementing and sustaining continuity of care. Evidence Based Midwifery.

Conference paper: A conference paper may be published as an article as well as be presented at a conference or within the conference proceedings.

- Example: Deeny, K., Clyne, W., Pezaro, S., and Kneafsey, S. (2017). Commissioning for compassion: the perceptions of healthcare commissioners about commissioning for positive staff experience. European Health Psychologist: 604–604.

Report: A report may be commissioned or produced as part of a research project. Rather than this being a scientific article as such, it is more of a detailed summary or overview of the work.

- Example: Royal College of Midwives. (2018). Safe places? Workplace support for those experiencing domestic abuse.

In thinking about exactly *what* to publish it is useful to think and plan ahead. In relation to a particular piece of work you have done, you also may consider why you want to publish it? For example, do you want to change something or have your evidence-based recommendations read by a group of people in particular? Once you decide this you can go ahead and think about your audience. That is, who you want to read your work or who you need to read your work in order to make change happen. In this sense, you can then think about what journals or articles your desired audience is reading and therefore plan as to how you will reach them yourself.

It is unusual for an author to publish alone. So, you will need to consider who you will author the publication with and why? This is crucial as the credit for a particular discovery or creation has a tremendous impact on people's lives. Whilst it is great to work with other midwives, different disciplines and authors can bring new ideas and perspectives. Who do you need on board to address all of the issues involved? In deciding who has contributed significantly enough to have a role in authorship it may be useful to consult the CRediT contributor role taxonomy as outlined by Brand et al. (2015) in Table 7.2.

Many publishers will request a CRediT author statement to be published alongside the work to ascertain which author contributed to what. If collaborators do not fall into any of these author roles, it may instead be pertinent to acknowledge or thank them for their particular insights or contributions elsewhere in the publication. In any case, it will be important to recognise the role of everyone involved, including funders.

TABLE 7.2 CRediT taxonomy.

Term	Definition
Conceptualisation	Ideas: formulation or evolution of overarching research goals and aims
Methodology	Development or design of methodology; creation of models
Software	Programming, software development; designing computer programs; implementation of the computer code and supporting algorithms; testing of existing code components
Validation	Verification, whether as a part of the activity or separate, of the overall replication/reproducibility of results/experiments and other research outputs
Formal analysis	Application of statistical, mathematical, computational or other formal techniques to analyse or synthesise study data
Investigation	Conducting a research and investigation process, specifically performing the experiments, or data/evidence collection
Resources	Provision of study materials, reagents, materials, patients, laboratory samples, animals, instrumentation, computing resources or other analysis tools
Data curation	Management activities to annotate (produce metadata), scrub data and maintain research data (including software code, where it is necessary for interpreting the data itself) for initial use and later reuse
Writing – original draft	Preparation, creation and/or presentation of the published work, specifically writing the initial draft (including substantive translation)
Writing – review & editing	Preparation, creation and/or presentation of the published work by those from the original research group, specifically critical review, commentary, or revision – including pre- or post-publication stages
Visualisation	Preparation, creation and/or presentation of the published work, specifically visualisation/data presentation
Supervision	Oversight and leadership responsibility for the research activity planning and execution, including mentorship external to the core team
Project administration	Management and coordination responsibility for the research activity planning and execution
Funding acquisition	Acquisition of the financial support for the project leading to this publication

Source: Brand et al., 2015 / John Wiley & Sons.

If you are considering publishing your work in a peer reviewed journal, there are several factors to consider. Firstly, if you want to publish the results of primary research, a respected journal will require you to have ethical approval for the work you have undertaken and a certification ID to prove it. Ethical approval is crucial in all cases (whether you intend to publish or not), and you will always need to declare this in a journal publication. You may also need to seek permission to publish results e.g. where they may relate to sensitive data from your organisation.

When determining which academic journal to publish your work in, and after deciding upon the audience you want to reach, you should consider where other respected authors in your field (or another field) publish. It is also worth considering which journals the authors you cite in your work are publishing in, as this may guide you to which journal may be most suited to your own work. Once you land on a potential target journal, it is important to consider whether you can meet their author guidelines for publication and whether you can publish without paying article processing fees (unless you have funds for this) which permit your work to be freely accessible to all once published (best practice!). Also of note, authors from certain countries may be eligible for fee waivers for publishing their work open access through efforts to decolonise research publications and raise the voices of academic researchers in underrepresented parts of the world– so it's worth checking!

Journal metrics in general can be a useful source of data with which to inform your decisions on where to publish. Yet many journal metrics can be confusing to navigate. For example, what exactly is an impact factor? Well, a journal's impact factor is based on a two-year period and is calculated by dividing the number of times its articles were cited by the number of articles that were citable in the journal. Very few journals have an impact factor of 10 or higher. In fact, most journals have an impact factor equal to or greater than 1. If a journal's impact factor is higher than 2 then it's in the 40% club. Yet it is important to note that different research areas have individual ranges to consider. There is also a debate around whether a journal's impact factor really matters. Does this 'impact' really translate into meaningful change?

The SCImago Journal ranking is another source you may wish to use when deciding which journal is 'best' to publish your work in. SCImago is a ranking tool and is calculated based upon the scientific influence of scholarly journals. This is measured by accounting for both the number of citations received by a journal and the reported prestige of the journals from where the citations come. The numeric value given indicates the average number of weighted citations received during a selected year per document published by the journal during the previous three years. A weighted citation includes the ratio of total citations received by the output, and the total citations that would be expected based on the average in the subject field. Each subject category of journals is divided into four quartiles (Q1, Q2, Q3, Q4). Q1 is occupied by the top 25% of journals in the list. Q2 is occupied by journals in the 25–50% group. Q3 is occupied by journals in the 50–75% group. Q4 is occupied by journals in the 75–100% group. In scoping out potential target journals it will be important to manage expectations. Consider whether your article matches your ambitions for publication. For example, if you have a small evaluation study to publish, you may want to aim for a Q3 or Q4 journal at the lower end of the spectrum, rather than a Q1 or Q2 journal at the higher end of the spectrum.

A journal's 'Citescore' relates to the number of citations received by a journal in one year to documents published in the three previous years. This number is then divided by the number of documents indexed in Scopus published in those same three years. A journal's citation count per paper divided by the citation potential in its subject area is known as it's source normalised impact per paper (SNIP) calculation. A journal's number of articles (h) which have received at least h citations is known as the journal's h index. This number largely relates to productivity and impact in science. The h Index is also applicable to individuals, institutions and countries. So, each academic who publishes will also have an h index which will grow over time (e.g. if an author's total article count is 33, yet 18 of these articles are cited at least 18 times, this would result in an h index of 18). Alongside such metrics, the following website resources may also help you in identifying the most appropriate journal in your publishing journey:

- www.scimagojr.com
- http://www.v2.sherpa.ac.uk/romeo
- http://www.jane.biosemantics.org (Ask Jane)
- https://doaj.org

Whatever the type of research or project you are planning to publish, it is important to consider whether there are associated reporting guidelines you could use to strengthen the publication of your work and ensure that it aligns with other publications of that type within the literature. Many journals will request the use of a reporting guideline, yet some won't. A reporting guideline lists the minimum set of items (usually as a checklist) that should be included in a research report to provide a clear and transparent account of what was done and what was found (Altman and Simera 2014). If you choose to use a reporting guideline to guide the reporting of your work, then make sure you cite which guideline you have used. Equally, it will be important to adhere to the guidelines you cite (reviewers and editors do check!). To evidence this adherence, you can add the checklist as an appendix to the report quoting exactly where in the document each item has been included. In Table 7.3, we list the main reporting guidelines available for you to peruse in relation to the type of study they apply to:

Before you submit your article for publication, you will also want to think about how people will locate your final article in order to read it. To stand out and be found or 'searchable' you will need to identify a strong article title and keywords. An article is more likely to be identified as relevant if its title contains key search terms and provides a clear description of the study and/or its findings. Overall, longer titles which use colons and acronyms, describe the study design in some way and avoid reference to any one specific country may be more successful in terms of being found and cited (Habibzadeh and Yadollahie 2010).

The chosen keywords should accurately represent the content of your manuscript and study. It is useful to ascertain what other authors in the field of

TABLE 7.3   Quality appraisal tools.

Guideline	Study type	Key elements	Observations
CONSORT (Schulz et al. 2010)	Randomised trials	25-item checklist, flow diagram	Extensions available for trial designs outside the most common; individually randomised, two group and parallel. Extensions available for additional designs
STROBE (Von Elm et al. 2014)	Observational studies	22-item checklist	Extensions available for study designs outside the most common; Cohort, case-control and cross-sectional
CHEERS (Husereau et al. 2013)	Evaluations	24-item checklist	Can be used with any form of economic evaluation (some may be named as cost-benefit analyses)
PRISMA (Moher et al. 2009)	Systematic reviews and meta-analyses	27-item checklist, flow diagram	PRISMA-P available for systematic review protocols PRISMA-ScR, available for reporting scoping reviews http://www.prisma-statement.org
MOOSE checklist (Stroup et al. 2000)	Meta-analyses of observational studies	35-item checklist	Refers to the Newcastle-Ottawa Scale for assessing the quality of non-randomised studies, a method of rating each observational study in your meta-analysis
CARE (Gagnier et al. 2012)	Case reports	13-item checklist	Examples offered via http://www.care-statement.org/checklist
SRQR (O'Brien et al. 2014) and COREQ (Tong et al. 2007)	Qualitative research	21-item checklist	Useful for interviews and focus group reporting
SQUIRE (Goodman et al. 2016)	Quality improvement	18-item checklist	Examples provided via http://www.squire-statement.org

midwifery are using as keywords. Yet, if it is not exclusively midwives you are looking to engage then other keywords may also be selected as being relevant. For example, in publishing work on the midwifery workforce, keywords relating to occupational health and human resources may also be relevant in engaging relevant professionals outside of the discipline. You could usefully search for the title of your manuscript in databases or simply Google Scholar prior to submitting it. This will help you to determine which keywords and other relevant studies are being identified with the words included. Would your article come up in a systematic search with its title? To assist you in answering this question, you can also identify terms and subject headings via a variety of subject databases. Ask a librarian to aid you in this task if you can.

Once your work is published (by the way... hurrah! Congratulations! ... this is not an easy nor a quick process) it is important to celebrate and share your work. Before you do this, check the journal's embargo period (if any) and any other publishing agreements in place. You may not be permitted to share the entire published PDF online. Yet there will certainly be links and other excerpts you will be able to shout about. You may first make your professional colleagues aware via email as you direct them to where they can read your latest publication. Yet evidence suggests that by sharing via social media, you will improve your reach and citation scores more significantly (Luc et al. 2021). See how we do this as academics by following us online (https://www.linktr.ee/SallyPezaro). Social media may also be a good place where you can highlight your work to key people/stakeholders (e.g. politicians) by tagging them in your social media posts about your work. You may also sign up for an ORCID (www.orcid.org) to uniquely identify yourself as an author of scholarly outputs and communication. Whilst you can share your findings and results at conferences and on personal blogs (e.g. http://sallypezaro.wordpress.com), it is best to do this only once the work is published in full.

We wish you all the best in navigating the somewhat rocky road of academic publishing, and we finish this section by leaving you with our top tips for publishing in peer reviewed journals:

- Don't slice projects – One strong and highly cited paper is better than many weaker ones that no-one ever cites
- Follow author and reporting guidelines thoroughly
- Check whether the methodology and methods are appropriate to answer the research question (The question should drive the study design)
- Don't simply write, 'to the best of our knowledge, nothing has been published in the field' unless you are really sure this is true – (a quick Google search by an editor or reviewer is all that is needed to make you look pretty silly).
- Provide a detailed point by point response to peer reviewers when revising a manuscript (you don't have to agree with everything a reviewer suggests, but you need to be really clear on the reasons why you don't in any rebuttal)
- References should be as recent as possible – Preferably some from the target journal
- Avoid complex 'flowery' language. Be concise and scientific.
- All research has limitations. It is important to explain what the limitations of a study might be beyond sample size and geographic location
- Aim for a strong 'light bulb' conclusion (don't just regurgitate what you have said)
- Be clear about your contribution to new knowledge
- Remember, 'data' are plural, so you need to write that the 'data were' rather than the 'data was' and check for this 'tense' issue throughout.

USING EVIDENCE TO INFORM PRACTICE

Finding all of the literature there is on a topic is well worth doing. However, this can be a long and systematic process, all of which we cannot cover within the confines of this book. Nevertheless, you can find out more on how to search the literature via my student tips blog pages (`http://sallypezaro.wordpress.com/category/student-tips`). You can also contact your organisation's librarian or library services to see what you have access to in terms of databases and literature search services. At a basic level, you can also browse academic search engines such as SCOPUS or PubMed to see indexed research on particular topics. Why not try to join some academic research groups too. Much of the time, the latest research articles are cascaded in these groups via email or shared via social media (see Chapter 2 on finding your community).

Once we find the literature, how do we know which evidence to use to inform our practice? After all, some articles will offer higher quality evidence than others. To help you decide, you will need to appraise the quality of evidence you find. The purpose of this quality appraisal is to identify the strengths and limitations of the studies you draw from (Porritt et al. 2014). In your quality appraisal, you may plan to establish the validity of the research you find (e.g. how true are the findings presented? Have the concepts been accurately measured? Would the findings be replicable in different contexts?). You may also plan to assess the risk of bias in each of the studies you find. In this sense, you would be asking whether the methods used in the study can be trusted to provide accurate results. Biases may be mitigated through randomisation, blinding and accurate reporting among other things. There are several biases to think about as listed in Table 7.4.

There are several quality appraisal tools to help you in this task. Planning which tool to use in appraising the quality of the articles you will find is important, as the chosen tool must be suited to appraising the types of articles you think you might find. There are several to choose from as outlined in more detail by Page et al. (2018) and Majid and Vanstone (2018) including:

- The GRADE-CERQual (Confidence in Evidence from Reviews of Qualitative research)
- GRADE (Grading of Recommendations Assessment, Development and Evaluation)

TABLE 7.4   Common biases.

Bias type	Explanation
Selection bias	Also known as allocation bias. Poor sample selection procedures result in non-representative samples.
Performance bias	Results in differences between groups in the care received
Detection bias/ measurement bias	Arises when outcomes are assessed differently for treatment and control groups
Attrition bias	Refers to differences in losses of subjects between groups

- Critical Appraisal Skills Programme (CASP)
- Evaluation Tool for Qualitative Studies (ETQS)
- The Mixed Methods Appraisal Tool (MMAT)
- CEBM: Centre for Evidence-Based Medicine (Oxford, UK)
- JBI (Joanna Briggs Institute) Critical Appraisal Tools Checklists provided for a range of study types and designs.
- Jadad scale for reporting randomised controlled trials
- McMaster Critical Review Form – For quantitative Studies
- Newcastle-Ottawa Scale (NOS) – A tool for assessing the quality of non-randomised studies, including case control and cohort studies.
- Cochrane Collaboration's tool for assessing risk of bias

These tools will typically include checklists, questions and scoring systems to guide you in garnering a final judgement on whether the research presented is of higher or lower quality. The higher the quality, the more likely you may be to include it in your practice and local guidelines. Overall, it will be most important to ensure that the tool you choose is the most appropriate for the types of research you will appraise, as some tools are better used for certain types of studies (e.g. qualitative, quantitative or mixed methods).

Below, we present one example of a tool for appraising the quality of qualitative research and one for the quality appraisal of quantitative research. Whilst you may use these more formally in your academic work, you may also use the questions included in your everyday practice to make swift assessments in relation to research.

Critical Appraisal of Quantitative Evidence: A Checklist from JBI

1. Is the assignment to treatment groups truly random?
2. Are participants blind to treatment allocation?
3. Is allocation to treatment groups concealed from the allocator?
4. Are the outcomes of people who withdrew described and included in the analysis?
5. Are those assessing the outcomes blind to the treatment allocation?
6. Are the control and treatment groups comparable at entry?
7. Are groups treated identically other than for the named interventions?
8. Are outcomes measured in the same way for all groups?
9. Are outcomes measured in a reliable way?
10. Is appropriate statistical analysis used?

Critical Appraisal of Qualitative Evidence: A Checklist from JBI

1. There is congruity between the stated philosophical perspective and the research methodology.
2. There is congruity between the research methodology and the research question or objectives.

3. There is congruity between the research methodology and the methods used to collect data.

4. There is congruity between the research methodology and the representation and analysis of data.

5. There is congruence between the research methodology and the interpretation of results.

6. There is a declaration of the researcher's cultural or theoretical orientation.

7. The influence of the researcher on the research, and vice versa, is addressed.

8. There is representation of participants and their voices.

9. There is ethical approval by an appropriate body.

10. There is a relationship between the conclusions of the study and the analysis or interpretation of the data.

Each of these tools has a maximum score of 10 available. Following their application, a higher score would be indicative of a higher quality piece of research, whilst a lower score would be indicative of a lower quality piece of research. You may also need to consider how feasible and/or cost-effective it might be to implement a study's findings in practice. Always consider the implications of any new change proposed in practice.

As well as there being a large time lapse between evidence cascading down to influence clinical practice, we recognised that there was also a large gap between research and educational practice (see Figure 7.1).

There is a need to ensure that future midwives and nurses are leading in research and evidence-based practice globally. The WHO has set its fourth priority area as promoting evidence-based practice and innovation, as evidence-based practice is every nurse's and midwife's concern and should be enabled by means of education, research, leadership and access to evidence sources (World Health Organisation 2015). Yet the management of the teaching–research nexus in practice can be complex. Significant evidence to practice gaps in the delivery of increasingly complex care exist but may be filled via RIT (Pezaro et al. 2022a). Essentially, there is a need to enhance the effective application of research into curricula.

Research and evidence have been used to inform and enhance clinical practice throughout history. Combining research and teaching activity within universities

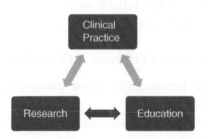

FIGURE 7.1   Relationship between practice, research and education.

is a relatively recent construct, which only began to develop in the early nineteenth century. According to Griffiths (2004) teaching may presently be;

- 'Research led' – The curriculum is structured around subject content (research findings); the emphasis is on understanding research findings rather than research processes.
- 'Research orientated' – The curriculum places emphasis as much on understanding the processes by which knowledge is produced in the field as on learning the knowledge that has been achieved.
- 'Research-based' in the sense that the curriculum is largely designed around inquiry-based activities.
- 'Research-informed' in the sense that it draws consciously on systematic inquiry into the teaching and learning process itself.

'Research-tutored' teaching also emphasises learning focused on students writing and discussing research publications (Healey 2005). Yet the Universitas 21 global network has declared that universities of the twenty-first century must now work together to foster RIT(see the beginning of this chapter for definitions). Through this call came the co-creation of the Research Inspired Online/Offline Teaching (RIOT) Framework (Pezaro et al. 2022a) (outlined in Figure 7.2) and aims to go beyond 'Tick Box' exercises in merely ensuring that the basics are met.

Co-creators suggested that this framework may be used as a 'benchmark of expectations'. Co-creators added the phrase 'Online/Offline' to emphasise its applicability in both realms of teaching. The framework's name was considered to form an acronym-as-analogy, which worked aptly to describe the positive disruption (RIOT) which co-creators anticipated this framework might bring. It is intended as a universal tool for both analysis and reflection. It is aimed at those looking to engage in 'research inspired teaching' and is offered to provide a more consensual standpoint on what it constitutes.

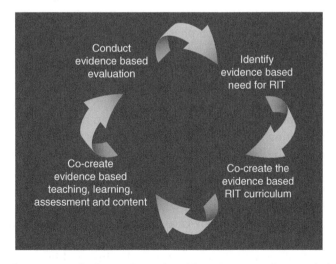

FIGURE 7.2   RIOT Framework. *Source*: Reproduced from Pezaro et al., 2022 / with permission of ELSEVIER.

Co-creators of this framework reflected that:

> *Those who engage with the RIOT framework are invited to embrace academic freedom, where both the educator and the self-actuated learner are entrusted and empowered to move away from inflexible learning structures and apply more individualised approaches.*
>
> *Being positively disruptive in replacing established models, paradigms, innovations and systems with improved ones is encouraged.*

The 10 Core Principles of the RIOT Framework include:

1. Establishment of multilateral relationships between teaching and research activities
2. Evidence-based decision-making
3. Academic freedom
4. Innovation
5. Positive disruption
6. Bridging between research centres and schools in HEIs
7. Authenticity
8. Maintaining the authority to teach through scholarly activities, research and/ or practice
9. Resulting 'Real world' impact
10. Co-creation

Whilst these core principles may seem exciting and pioneering for practice, there is also a need to know how the framework may be applied in a practical sense. Accordingly, co-creators explored how the four phases of the RIOT framework may be thought about and what might be done in each phase (Table 7.5).

Evidence-based decision-making must be applied to pedagogical approaches and subject materials at every level to avoid the delivery of outdated teaching, uninformed by contemporary evidence and/or optimal teaching approaches. Students are better enriched when teaching, scholarship, research and/or professional practice are linked together. RIT may inspire students to embrace careers in midwifery/nursing research and thus align in meeting the 'Global strategic directions for nursing and midwifery 2021–2025' to increase the proportion and authority of future midwives and nurses in senior academic positions. We would love to hear about how you are using the RIOT framework in your own practice (see the activity at the end of this chapter).

Ultimately, it will be crucial for midwives to use the best available evidence to inform their practice throughout their careers. We hope that this chapter has given you a broad introduction on how you might ensure your own practice is evidence informed. This book along with its content was also inspired by research as is illustrated by our real-life experiences. Living a research inspired life is something of a habit for us. We hope it becomes the same way for you because research and evidence are essentially what can change the world.

TABLE 7.5 The four phases of the RIOT framework.

Phase one: identify evidence-based need for RIT	Need to 'reflect on why we need this (RIT) on a societal level, or for the public good'
	The evidence-based need for RIT should be defined and communicated from the outset
	Enquire as to which specific gaps in knowledge exist and need to be filled
Phase two: co-create the evidence-based RIT curriculum	Co-creators reflected that curriculum designers 'need to be co-creating with the people who it will impact' in order to 'avoid a "doing to" approach'
	There is a need for co-creation to 'ensure all stakeholders are part of it', bringing their own evidence base, perspectives and expertise into curriculum design
	Explore the ways in which research centres might use their leverage
	Identify key expertise early on to engage them in co-creating RIT curriculums
	Identify and enquire as to how the programme or course of study should flow, and what topics it may cover
	Healthcare services may evidence a need for new subject specific skills to be included for their future workforce. This may be updated on a regular basis
Phase three: co-create evidence-based teaching, learning, assessment and content	Need to co-create evidence-based teaching, learning and assessment activities, and content to 'provide students with the opportunity of being involved in the design of learning and formative assessment through their learning journey'.
	Important to ensure that all teaching, learning and assessment activities and content are inspired by evidence gathered via research
	Educators engaging in RIT should seek to gain inspiration from both pedagogical and subject specific sources of evidence
	Any research inspired teaching, learning and assessment activities should be 'conceptually meaningful to engaging students' (e.g. increasing student's exposure to research centres and their activities through buddying systems, mentorship, research internships and secondments in order to understand what researchers do and engage and inspire them)
	Important to bridge schools, faculties and research centres in Higher Education Institutions (HEIs) and develop multilateral relationships between teaching and research activities
	An inspiring space must also be co-created for research, along with seminar and conference opportunities for the sharing of it
	All students 'need to develop research skills' in order to engage in any meaningful inquiries and apply evidence to practice. (It is also important for students to both 'consume' and 'do' research)
	Educators should be encouraged to undertake activities which maintain their authority to teach

(Continued)

TABLE 7.5   (Continued)

Phase four: conduct evidence-based evaluation	In conducting evidence-based evaluations of RIT, both educators and students may identify the ways in which they can usefully explore, evaluate, improve, refine and examine the effectiveness and replicability of it empirically
	What has or has not taken place? What new knowledge has been co-created? What impact?
	Conducting an evidence-based evaluation may also provide confirmation of the need for future RIT in subsequent student populations, thus prompting a return to phase one of the RIOT framework
	Educational content, along with any teaching, learning and assessment activities may be updated, augmented, refined and adapted in response to any new evidence available, and in readiness for the delivery of future RIT (teaching may indeed inspire further research)

IN CONVERSATION (KAREN AND SALLY SHARE INSIGHT FROM THEIR ACADEMIC CAREER JOURNEY)

KM   Did you always know you wanted to be academic?

SP   No, I didn't do well at school. I was too busy having fun with friends. It was only really once I went to university and realised what academia was really all about and what I could achieve in applying it myself. I still don't find academia 'easy' necessarily. But I do now see it more as a motivating and intriguing strategic puzzle in need of constant resolve. Once you know the basic rules, things become a lot simpler. Nevertheless, I am challenging my brain every day.

KM   Same here. My GCSE grades were ok, my A-levels less so and stumbled into an undergraduate degree at 19 years old studying sports where I spent more time playing than studying. I came back to university later in life once I had my children following several years working in health and well-being. I'd always been interested in psychology and used various psychological techniques in my job as a health coach without really understanding why or where they came from. So, following redundancy, I went back to study psychology and found that when you are interested and passionate about something, motivation to study and curiosity about the topic takes a life of its own. What was supposed to be a one year top up of my knowledge turned into three postgraduate degrees, a PhD and a Chartership with the British Psychological Society. How did you find coming back to studying after your career in practice? And what motivated you to make that change?

SP   Like many clinicians I suppose, I felt as if I was behind other academics who had come straight from undergraduate study to master's and PhDs. Those years in clinical practice didn't seem to count for much at first. Neither did my undergraduate degree in the arts.

The thought of going back into clinical practice after what I had been through was not appealing to me, though I did the odd clinical shift here and there. I needed a new challenge, and an opportunity to make sense of everything from an academic perspective. I am so glad I won a studentship to complete my PhD. I really believe I am thriving more now than I ever would have done if I had not had that opportunity.

KM Academia has a bit of an image that only certain types of people can become academics but that simply isn't true. Often those of us who come from a non-traditional academic background hide our journeys through fear of being outed as a fraud which perpetuates the image of academia as an ivory tower even further. I hope sharing our journeys shows that your background, previous education experience or chosen discipline doesn't need to hold you back.

SP Indeed, and I hope people draw strength from us if they are looking to make that change.

Activity – Using the RIOT Framework in Practice

In this chapter, we have introduced you to the RIOT framework in the hope that it would embolden you to engage in 'research inspired teaching' – mapping research and education together for the benefit of both. Using the RIOT framework as a guide, co-create a small session in your local area (either with colleagues or students). We would love to hear about how this framework is being used in practice. If you can, please contribute to ongoing impact data collection and tell us how you have used this framework in practice (sally.pezaro@coventry.ac.uk).

CHAPTER 8

Leading with Impact

INTRO TO CHAPTER

Some of you reading this book may already be in a formal leadership position, others may be only just starting out on their midwifery journey so leadership may not be something you have considered yet, and others still may feel that formal leadership is not something that you want for your career. Regardless of where you fit in those descriptions, leadership at work affects us all either through being the person with formal responsibility or being those followers in their charge. But as we discuss within this chapter, we have the capacity to display leadership in our everyday interactions, at every level. Therefore, we hope this section is of benefit to everyone regardless of how they see leadership in their midwifery journey. We will discuss useful theories of leadership that can help develop the midwifery leaders of the future and help shape your own leadership practice. In addition, we will explore how small actions of leadership everyday have the potential to make a change from the ground up.

WHAT IS A LEADER?

Leadership is one of the most widely debated but least clearly understood concepts within business and management studies. There are close to as many definitions of a leader or leadership as there are researchers studying it. Traditionally, leadership was thought of in terms of people in positions of power, who used that power and authority to influence others. However, the way we think about leadership has changed over recent decades. It is less about the person in a certain position in an organisation and what they do, and more about the process of influencing others towards a commonly held goal. By opening out the definition of leadership towards the process extends the possibility of a leader

Surviving and Thriving in Midwifery, First Edition. Sally Pezaro and Karen Maher.
© 2025 John Wiley & Sons Ltd. Published 2025 by John Wiley & Sons Ltd.

not only being in a formal leadership position but also to others within a team who stimulate, move and energise their teammates towards their objectives.

Leadership is a social action between two or more people. Followers allow themselves to be led, either willingly or unwillingly dependent upon the situation. The relationship between the leader and their followers can be instrumental in the success or otherwise of any attempt towards achieving work goals. Traditional top-down command and control styles of leadership, seen within the military as an example, are ineffective in many workplaces including midwifery. Participative approaches to leadership allow followers to have a voice, building trust and psychological safety; concepts we have touched on throughout this book which are important for successful leadership. Later in this chapter, we will explore ways of building psychological safety within your own teams.

There are a vast number of different theories and models of leadership within the academic literature, and it is impossible to cover them all within this chapter. As you go through the chapter you will notice that we have chosen to focus on a few key theories that we feel have the greatest potential to shape the midwifery leaders the profession needs. Because we are viewing leadership as a social process rather than a position of formal authority, our definition of a leader for the purposes of this section is:

> *a person who influences, inspires, supports and encourages a group of people and constantly works to achieve goals (Bekhruz 2022, p. 136)*

As you will see later in this chapter, this definition allows for emergent and informal leadership behaviours and provides the opportunity for all midwives to be leaders in their own way.

But it is not all about the leader. Without followers, there are no leaders, and there is a power in being the first follower; the one that sees the potential in the message someone is selling. Without the first follower, there is only a passionate person talking to themselves. Great ideas need people to catch them. So don't be afraid to be the first follower when you see the potential of something new put forward by someone in your team.

WHAT KIND OF LEADER WILL YOU BE?

Before you move forward in your leadership journey, it will be important to reflect on what kind of leader you might be to get the best performance out of those who follow you. Literature suggests the existence of three major mechanisms that shape collegial characteristics and influence performance by affecting:

1. their ability to perform, including use of their knowledge, skills and abilities.
2. their motivation (e.g. through compensation and incentives) which influences staff attitudes by affecting their motivation, commitment and satisfaction.
3. their opportunity to perform, or how their involvement and job design may reduce turnover and absenteeism.

(Appelbaum et al. 2000; Katou and Budhwar 2010)

These components may be leveraged by leaders to enhance performance. In what ways does or could the midwifery workplace leverage these mechanisms to make the most of staff? How are midwives motivated, given opportunities and how are their knowledge, skills and abilities best utilised? As a leader, these are the things you will need to consider, whereby policies and practices are shaped to maximise opportunities in this regard.

Leadership will always be about turning overarching (rather than personal) visions into practice (we will take you through this in Chapter 9). Yet how do you forge such a vision to communicate?

According to Collins and Porras (1991), vision consists of a guiding philosophy (rooted in organisational core beliefs and purpose) and a tangible image (engaging and descriptive to focus efforts on achieving the shared future imagined). In this sense, we can go through the following formula to identify the vision we need to communicate as leaders ourselves.

- Core values + Core purpose = Guiding philosophy
- Mission + Tangible vision = Tangible image
- Guiding philosophy + Tangible image = Vision

Think back to when you made your vision statement or statement of purpose in Chapter 2. In deciding the kind of leader you might be, it will first be important to discover what your purpose might be as a leader. When doing this gather in a small group of a few peers and grapple with the following three questions posed by Craig and Snook (2014):

- What did you especially love doing when you were a child before the world told you what you should or shouldn't like or do? Describe a moment and how it made you feel.
- Explain two of your most challenging life experiences. How have they shaped you?
- What do you enjoy doing in your life now that helps you 'sing your song'?

After this exercise, you may wish to go back and amend or add to the vision statement or the statement of purpose in Chapter 2. That's fine. This is, after all, a progressive and continuous journey of insight and learning.

One of the popular theories of leadership, which still has traction today, focuses on the ways in which leaders share their vision and bring others along with them in the journey towards successful achievement. Transformational leadership theory (Bass 1985, 1997; Burns 1978) suggests that successful leaders build relationships with their followers around a common purpose where both parties are inspired, mobilised and grow as they move towards their goal. The leader becomes the role model for others, setting an example and challenging their followers in ways which see them motivated to go beyond self-interest and work towards a higher collective purpose. One key component of transformational leadership is that the actions of the leader serve both the leader and the followers so there is mutual benefit, not simply the use

TABLE 8.1 Theoretical components of transformational leadership.

Individualised consideration	The leader treats each follower on their own merits and seeks to develop followers through delegation of projects and coaching/mentoring
Intellectual stimulation	The leader encourages free thinking and emphasises reasoning before action is taken
Inspirational motivation	The leader creates an optimistic, clear, attainable vision of the future thus encouraging others to raise their expectations
Idealised influence	The leader makes personal sacrifices, takes responsibility for their actions, shares any glory and shows great determination

of charm to wield power in self-interest. Bass (1985) puts forward four components of transformational leadership which identify behaviours transformational leaders exhibit as outlined in Table 8.1. Are there ways in which you display these components? Are there any midwives in your network that model these components? If so, think about how their teams respond.

You can become more effective as a leader by critically reflecting on your leadership style, approach and the organisational context in which you operate. For example, how do you share your vision with those in your team? How do you reward and motivate those around you? Is it contingent on certain actions or do you adjust how you motivate based upon the needs of everyone? How do you model the behaviour you wish to see in others? To grow as a more effective leader, you may need to adapt your leadership style to different situations. Whilst I (Sally) have been fortunate enough to have completed an MSc in Healthcare Leadership, a postgraduate diploma in Global Leadership and leadership training via the Oxford Executive Leadership Programme in the Saïd Business School at the University of Oxford, as midwives, we may not always receive such leadership training and education. However, there are lots of resources available to help develop your leadership potential, why not reach out to see what is available in your part of the world?

Through our reflection we can notice when our behaviours match with our vision. The more aligned our behaviours are with our vision and values the more authentic our leadership becomes. Authentic leadership (Avolio and Gardner 2005) is where the leader remains true to their values and beliefs and acts in a way that is consistent with those values and beliefs. Through self-awareness and self-regulated positive behaviours, authentic leaders build positive relationships with their followers. It is important to note that Avolio and Gardner's definition of authentic leadership encompasses a positive moral perspective. Other scholars do not make this distinction and thus see the possibility for a leader to be authentically true to nefarious or self-serving values. However, in our aim of sharing leadership theory which has benefits for midwifery, Avolio and Gardner's approach allows us to explore the ways in which personal insight can influence positive relationships for the benefit of the leader, the team and wider midwifery. Table 8.2 outlines the four components of authentic leadership proposed by Avolio and Gardner. As you read through them, consider whether you recognise leaders in your organisation or that you have worked

TABLE 8.2 Theoretical components of authentic leadership.

Self-awareness	Being aware of motives, emotions, traits that guide behaviour. An honest and accurate view of one's own strengths and weaknesses. Reflecting on actions and outcomes to gain insight
Unbiased/balanced processing of information	Being able to consider others' thoughts and views fairly and considerately whilst sharing one's own
Internalised moral perspective	Having an ethical foundation and positive moral framework shaping values and beliefs
Relational transparency	Being able to present one's true self to others to create relationships based on trust, and encouraging others to do the same

with previously displaying authentic leadership behaviours described? How did/do those leaders make you feel as a follower?

WE ARE ALL LEADERS

Whilst we may think of our leaders as those with a high-powered position or role, we are all leaders in practice, displaying our own leadership behaviours and cultivating our abilities to lead through our everyday activities and behaviours. We will discuss this later on in the chapter, but it is also important to remember that with leadership comes power, and with power comes responsibility. Yukl (2013) presents seven distinct forms of power. These are both positional and personal and can be broadly described as follows:

Positional power – **Can weaken satisfaction, performance and commitment of followers**

1. **Legitimate power:** This is the idea that you have power by virtue of the position you are in. That is, you may be in a position to form guidance and policy. This form of power may be reinforced when followers adhere to the requests of those with positional power. Equally, this power can be exploited should a leader attempt to exercise power outside of their sphere of influence. However, this form of power can be weakened if it is perceived by followers that the position has not been given fairly.

2. **Reward power:** In this, the leader has the power to bestow rewards upon followers (e.g. through pay, incentives, rewarding work tasks) to incentivise performance. This power may be rebalanced when followers are enabled feedback systems upon which leaders equally rely upon for their own pay and rewards.

3. **Coercive power:** This is essentially power derived from the threat or action of punishment and/or reprimand. These may compel followers to abide by the requests of the leader. However, legislation and unions may curtail coercive power somewhat.

4. **Information power:** The source of power here comes from having control over access to and distribution of information. Leaders may have access to information that their followers do not allowing them to select which information to share to appear more favourable. This form of power can be seen in those without a formal leadership role such as when working with student midwives in a supervisory way or if an individual's role requires them to collect/analyse information or data.

5. **Ecological power:** Here an individual has control over the physical work environment, technology, or structure of work tasks which has an indirect influence over others. So, an example of this could be a manager responsible for the allocation of shifts or duties on a given shift.

Personal power – **Creates a sense of trust**

6. **Expert power:** This is essentially where the leader is regarded as an expert in their field and therefore holds power in being recognised by followers as trustworthy and authoritative. Specialist knowledge is becoming increasingly more important in leadership as we find ourselves dealing with evermore complex phenomena. Expert power may also be seen in those without formal leadership positions.

7. **Referent power:** Through charisma and a distinctive leadership style, one can accumulate referent power as they in turn gain the admiration and respect of their followers. With this power, they may then influence, motivate, inspire and persuade their followers to both carry out tasks and execute certain agendas. When combined with expert power, leaders who can cultivate this may become a particularly formidable force in both organisations and professions alike. However, using referent power alone may not be enough over the long term as they may be perceived as lacking in substance and thus lose any respect initially gained.

Reflect: It is useful to reflect upon the types of power that are exercised both by yourself and in your midwifery teams and organisations. In your reflections ask yourself:

- Which policies and procedures constrain or promote the different types of power in your context?
- Which types of power do you hold as a leader?
- How will you avoid abusing this power in your particular context?
- Legitimate, expert and referent power may be utilised simultaneously to produce the most desirable outcomes – How might you foster this in practice? Consider both your peers and followers in this.

If you are already a leader by virtue of the job or position of power you hold, you may want to consider what approach you may take in leading from an organisational perspective. Farkas and Wetlaufer (1996) interviewed 160 chief executive officers and identified five standard approaches to such leadership. These are broadly described as:

The strategy approach: In this sense, the leader is more concerned about long-term strategy rather than short-term operational management. They are the overseers of an organisation and tend to spend more time engaging externally rather than internally.

The human assets approach: Unsurprisingly, this approach involves investment in people as the leader sets the values, attitudes and behaviours expected of those who are developed by the leader, who also engages predominantly in personnel matters above other things.

The expertise approach: This approach focuses on the leader cultivating and selecting expertise to gain competitive advantages in the field. They then focus on disseminating and building on this expertise internally.

The box approach: This is largely an approach dedicated to monitoring finances and cultures within an organisation. Through this approach, the leader develops policies and procedures that reinforce organisational expectations in terms of behaviour and performance.

The change approach: Innovation and reinvention lies at the heart of this approach, as leaders seek to motivate others in embracing change and continuous improvement.

One small thing: Much of the discussion so far has focused on a formalised idea of leadership. But what about the idea posed at the start of this section, that we are all leaders? Our everyday behaviour has the potential to exact change or make a difference to someone else, sometimes without us even knowing. Everyday leadership is where we make intentional choices to create better connections, communication and community where we work. This can include taking a moment to check in with the midwives on your ward during a busy shift to see how they are doing, making a conscious choice to respond calmly and positively even on a bad day (and perhaps when it isn't reciprocated), thinking outside the box and trying new ways of working rather than the ways things have always been done. Small acts can make a big difference because they can become contagious.

Traditional theories of leadership, including transformational and authentic leadership mentioned earlier in this section, focus on the relationship between the leader and the follower or the human capital required for competent leadership. But complexity leadership theory (CLT) (Uhl-Bien and Marion 2009) takes an alternative view, suggesting that everyday interactions between individuals within the workplace drive success rather than a single leader forging a path that others follow. Midwifery, and healthcare in general, is a complex and dynamic working environment. The social interactions that take place are multiple across hierarchies, disciplines and types of work task, often without a formal leader present. These everyday interactions have the potential to evolve new ways of working and innovative solutions to problems organically, rather than through a policy or process. Therefore, anyone within midwifery has the capacity and capability to lead and shape outcomes within their service. Through leveraging your social capital as you respond to everyday events and triggers at work, you become a catalyst for change.

Within CLT, the role of the formal leader within a complex work environment is to foster the necessary conditions that drive successful social interactions, which allows the small acts to become contagious. Leaders, whether individually or collectively, need to be aware of, engage with and harness the potential of the dynamic and complex midwifery context. According to Arena and Uhl-Bien (2016), this can be achieved by engaging in adaptive practices guided by adaptive principles as outlined in Tables 8.3 and 8.4. Depending upon the midwifery context in which you work, some of the

TABLE 8.3   Adaptive practices.

Practice	Practice description
Positive deviance	Problem-solving and community driven approach to enable the discovery of successful local behaviours and solutions. Exploration of new ways of working outside the norm, which has benefits to the way we do things around here
Liberating structures	Simple tools to enhance co-ordination, participation and trust in teams to creatively problem solve and develop new ideas
Design thinking	Consideration of tools which place humans at the heart of the thinking. Can we engineer out human error from the way we work?
Adaptive salons	Focus groups to encourage brainstorming around critical issues
Co-labs	Intensive ideas incubator experience where teams collaborate and compete to pitch ideas and solutions
Adaptive summits	Large group events to foster a community of change agents to co-create a way of working

Source: adapted from Arena and Uhl-Bien (2016).

TABLE 8.4   Adaptive principles.

Principle	Principle description
Start small	Think big but start small. Having a 'just get started' attitude where ideas are iteratively tested, shared and built upon
Find a friend	Building new ideas alongside new relationships is hard, so leverage relationships you already have as you evolve your ideas. Find local allies to test and develop ideas
Follow the energy	Link with existing ideas, strategies and advocates. Build momentum for each other's plans. Find ways to make passion flourish
Set boundaries	Proximity is essential to maintaining momentum. Initially, limit engagement to a group of natural networks, those you already interact with
Embrace the conflict	An idea must have fitness to be meaningful to an organisation. Fitness is strengthened through modification or an adaptive response to conflict. If someone rejects your idea, explore why and whether an adaptation can be made
Create network closure	Encouragement of the individuals within a network responsible for an idea to close around a sponsor for formal endorsement into the wider organisation

Source: adapted from Arena and Uhl-Bien (2016).

practices may be more difficult to implement than others. Only you will know your context well enough to determine how these can be applied and we have only provided suggestions within the descriptions.

Whilst we are all leaders in midwifery, Sally had the ultimate delight of meeting with Franka Cadee, a former President of the International Confederation of Midwives (ICM) to discuss how Franka has personally survived and thrived as an ICM midwifery leader. See their conversation below:

Sally   Hello Franka, thank you for meeting with me today. I was hoping that you might be able to draw on some of your experiences to give some insight into how you have personally survived and thrived in midwifery for the benefit of others trying to do the same.

Franka   Yes, I can. And it's in different ways, of course, because I have my hands-on midwifery work from the past, but I think it might be best just to do it in my ICM role.

Sally   Yes, please do.

Franka   Even though I do sit on the ground nationally, many organisations like in the UK are really struggling. But I do think that globally ICM is doing well, and I think that has been because we've also survived.

When I first came into ICM, I had to think in many ways also about the reputation of midwives in general. This kind of gender thing whereby, you know, we're looked upon as feeling sorry for ourselves or that we were only difficult. We had a lot of that when I first came in. Our partners in general had a lot of negative things to say about us; that we didn't have our things in order, that we complained a lot and that we basically felt like we were hard done by all the time. Felt very, very sorry for ourselves.

So, it's me, the board and the head office. We decided look, you know, we are just going to stand there and speak up and not make any excuses anymore. We're just gonna be there, unapologetic. So, we made a really firm decision. We will always speak, and I think at the table we actually in many ways became louder, but we also used a lot more evidence. So, we really said you know this is the evidence for midwifery. This is what midwives are for. This is what ICM is for.

Although it was very hard to begin with, I think it took about three to four years. Slowly, slowly, with the evidence, organisations changed. I do still get the comments that we are allowed and difficult... but now I get it more with respect. I get it with a smile, and I feel that in that way we're really thriving and I'm so pleased that we are because I think midwifery and the evidence from midwifery are becoming so strong.

Sally   That's amazing Franka, what else do you see changing in healthcare?

Franka   I think that in maternity care, I think the balance is changing. I also think that many of the other healthcare professionals feel that the balance is changing and is very much changing for midwifery care because it's prevention. The basis of it is so strong, especially in high-income countries. The low- and middle-income countries have always had a lot of **** come over them. But in the high-income countries... the UK and New Zealand, Canada, Germany, Denmark, Sweden, the Netherlands it's all about power and...there are a lot of ways in which I think organisations or other people within maternity care are trying to blame or push us down. Yet we are free, and I think it is because the power balance is changing. I think we're at the point of really changing the paradigm and when you are about to change the paradigm, you get a period of chaos and difficulty and pain.

Sally   So where does the ICM go from here?

Franka   I feel certainly at the ICM we're thriving. We're clear globally, we're clear where we're going and we're saying it in such a positive way, certainly financially. You know, we've trebled in size, we are much more able to communicate the message, we're much more visible. We're taken much more seriously. Organisations come to us nowadays to ask us to collaborate with us instead of the other way around. I think this has come at an opportune time because so many of our associations are having such a hard time.

I found it really hard to begin with. I found it really difficult to get these kinds of comments.

Sally   That midwives and the ICM were perceived as being 'difficult'?

Franka   Yes, at times it was very personal. You know, people looked at me at the table and they would say to me, *'you know, Franka midwives, you know, you're just so hard to work with. You're so angry all the time'*. And I think certainly my way, (And I think there would be many different ways) but my way has been to say, *'well, tell me more'*... *'How do you think we can make it better?'* and to be a bit more open and humbler and say, well, *'help me'!*... *'Help us!'* I think in that way we have made personal bonds with organisations and people in those organisations because, you know, you can say that you work well with other organisations, but it's always the people.

Sally   Indeed. So, in that way the ICM and yourself have really been able to thrive.

Franka   Yes, and we have come through a hard, a very hard period. Also, financially, five years ago we were rock bottom. We didn't know we would survive the next year. Now we are really financially doing extremely well, but we have to be very careful because you know, when you really grow, you have to make sure that you keep your team together, that you keep your eyes on the ball, that you can accept the change together, that you keep motivated together. It's a dangerous time in a way. But I do feel really proud of it. I really feel it's a huge change.

Sally   Yes, I definitely see the changes as well. A lot of what you were saying about the evidence being so strong and needing that evidence in order to invoke change was really powerful. It is also interesting to hear about how listening to other people and asking them to help you aided you in thriving. What were some of the changes you made in response to other people's advice?

Franka We started working more regionally with midwifery associations as we were told to, because I think before we were in a bit of confusion. We thought we were like a development aid organisation. Yet we're not a development aid organisation, we're a membership organisation and all the members are our members, and all our members need us in different ways.

In some countries, the members need us to help them to get organised as their maternal mortality is huge, whilst in other countries they are trying to keep the caesarean section rate down. It really, really varies from country to country. But what we were told is *'focus on your member associations. Listen to your members, be more diverse'*. That's one thing that we were really told be more diverse, have your board be more diverse.

I think we were quite Anglophone really and, in that way, we have really tried hard to, well, we focus more on our regions. So, we have regional meetings nowadays and we focus more on what each region needs. In many ways, our groups are smaller now and that is something that was very much said to us. *'Look, look at that. Look at your regions, listen to your members, be more open to diversity'*. And I think that that's something that we've worked on within the board and within the head office.

Another thing, our board, when I first started and still now, we have three European board members, which actually in respect to the rest of the world, Europe, population wise, it doesn't make sense that you have three. We have northern Europe, Central Europe, southern Europe and then you have Asia Pacific as one region. So, we decided to go to the WHO regions and make Europe one region. And I do feel that as a European person I was able to do that. I think because it is about my own region, so I was able to say, look, you know we need to go to one region being three regions is just not OK.

I do feel that moving away from the ICM using only three languages is a good thing. We have millions of, you know, thousands of languages, it's the colonial strength.

Another thing we're doing, and we haven't started that yet, but we will from the next training onwards, it's that at the moment working for the board is voluntary. But being able to work voluntarily all sounds very nice and humble, but you can only do it when you're in a privileged position to be able to afford your house. So, I can only afford this because my husband works and in many ways is supporting me. I get a little bit of an honorarium, but I hardly get anything. So, if I were a midwife in sub-Saharan Africa or in Southeast Asia and I was also the breadwinner, I would never be able to be the ICM President, even if I had the capacity or the competencies.

Sally Wow, that's really powerful to think about.

Franka Yeah, it's really something I've learned through ICM. I've always thought …Working voluntarily, whilst such a humble and wonderful thing to do, I do think we need to remember that when you work voluntarily, you can do that because you can afford to.

So, I've changed it that from next year onwards there will be a three-day kind of pay for the president, which means that someone coming from Southeast Asia or sub-Saharan Africa can afford to become the president because they'll be paid.

Interestingly, I was discussing this with the International Federation of Gynaecology and Obstetrics (FIGO), and I said that we had this issue and that they didn't understand at all. They were saying *well, 'what we do is voluntarily, we really believe that we should do it voluntarily'* and I didn't get it through to them to make them see, but yes, great that you're doing it voluntarily but do realise why you can do it voluntarily and we would never be able to get an African President in because nearly all the African midwives are breadwinners, they would never be able to afford to do this.

That is also why we don't get diverse presidents, we don't. We have had a few black presidents, but they've all been from the UK.

Sally Yeah. And it's interesting what you say about competence as well because offering these opportunities is one thing but having the capacity and the skill set to do it could be lacking in some geographical areas where access to education and training is lower.

Franka Yeah. Yeah, there is. I think that is a difficulty anyway, although at times it's also that we are not open to different ways of doing different things. We have a very kind of Western way and that is a really hard one when it comes to diversity and equality, this is really difficult because it's kind of like you know, it's like paternalism. You don't hardly see it. A fish doesn't see water.

Sally Indeed.

Franka I also think that we need leadership training for our board members, future board members and we are thinking of that and already doing it with the current board members and changing the whole way in which we're looking at competencies and really trying to steer on competencies because I think you know when you have a stronger head office, you really need a stronger board.

A board that is able to ask the right questions of that stronger head office. Having a governance system in place is also really useful when it can work as governance and when it can really govern and ask the right questions. But if that board doesn't have the competencies to do that, you get an organisation that goes out of balance.

Sally Absolutely. That would be really interesting to see in the next few years how that changes the dynamics within the board and also what the ICM can achieve or aim to achieve.

Franka   Yeah. Yeah, yeah...

Because at the moment, what I find, for example, there's one organisation. And I've tried really hard. I've worked so hard to get more midwives at the table, and I think it's one of the few times in my career when I've really, literally put my fist on the table with anger that I found that with their new governance structure, they just put in obstetricians all over the place. But no midwives, not out of bad will, by the way, not at all bad will, but just not seeing it.

Sally   Yes, utterly frustrating in any context.

Franka   Yeah, just overlooking it. And in the end, it really changed it. They managed, they put more midwives in place, but what is hard is that I now have to every month sit with those midwives to support them, to be able to say the right things at the table because we are often not trained well enough to be savvy enough to work within that system. And so, at times, you know, people don't come to meetings, and I think, uh, you know, I've tried so hard to get people here, but you know, you have to get people to the point that they realise why and the politics of it. So, we're really in a chicken and egg situation at times.

But you do have to just dare. You just have to dare and start it.

Sally   Absolutely. Do you think this is because some midwives do not feel valued enough to speak up?

Franka   Yep, I think that still exists. Yeah, I think it does. And I think that's the one that we really have to work on, and we do have our young leadership programmes but I do hope that trickles through and in general actually, I would love it that one day we'll make sure that we have a student on the board. I would love to have a client on the board too. Uh, but the first steps we're making now are opening it up a bit for the first time. Now we have the possibility of a non-midwife as a treasurer. I think again that is really great. It can be a midwife, but it doesn't have to be. And that means that we can be stronger, we can use the skills of others to thrive.

Asking for help, that's one thing I really feel that we've asked for help in an open, strong way. But when you do it that way people help.

Sally   Yeah. Well, it's like being humble and vulnerable in asking for help. But actually, it's the strongest thing to do.

Franka   Yeah, yeah. Yeah, I think it is. I certainly feel that as I see midwives globally, we have survived. We have now survived 100 years and that I think in many ways we're thriving. At the same time, I worry that what I do see on the ground is so much more complex and we have to really be real and realise that so many people are struggling in a big way. I'm pleased that at least globally, we're strong enough that we can possibly support midwives to pull themselves together because it's really hard, I found it extremely painful to see.

Sally   Yes, I see it too. Meeting people throughout the writing of this book and talking to people has been really eye opening. Do you have any top tips or lasting thoughts you could leave the readers of this book in terms of how you think they can survive and thrive in practice when it is so challenging out there?

Franka   One thing that has really helped me. Stay true to what you truly believe in so that you feel that you're doing the right thing. We must be able to look at ourselves in the mirror and think *'yes, this is OK'*. Stick to your guns and believe in yourself. Finally, I think it's important to find help, find others to go with you. You know often when we go to congresses and things like that, we say *'Oh yeah we're preaching through the converted'*. I've really come to realise that preaching to the converted is so important because we need to kind of like polish our souls, don't we? Every so often we need to kind of get energy again so that we can keep going.

Finding mates is important, finding partners, friends that will support you and that you can talk to, and even though they say the same as you, you feel strengthened, find help, find help. Don't think you have to do it alone. You're not alone. Midwives are not alone. We're a huge community really and a very special community.

I find it strengthens me enormously to know, you know, you. I'm seeing you here opposite me. It feels just great to be speaking to a midwife.

Sally   Indeed, the feeling is mutual, and in finding *'your people'* they can kind of validate the direction you're going in and what you're trying to achieve.

Franka   Yeah. Yeah, yeah. And that you will do your own thing. So, one person might do it with a woman. You're doing it with this book. You and I have had discussions about nurses, nurses and midwives and stuff like that. You can agree on certain things. You can differ. You can try to find the edges and you can still stand that together. And I'm so proud of you for doing this. It's so fantastic. And I couldn't do it. You can do it.

Sally   Wow, thank you! I am certainly trying to make an impact where I can as a midwife, and you know in doing what we both do for midwifery, whilst we don't catch babies physically, we are still midwives.

Franka   Yeah, absolutely. I felt that for a while. I thought I'm not allowed to say I'm a midwife. And then one day I thought, what am I talking about? Of course, I'm allowed to call myself a midwife. I really feel I am a midwife. You are a midwife.

Sally   Exactly. That's so true. And it runs throughout me. I don't think you could ever take the midwife out of me. It's who I am, and I thank you so much for giving your time and wisdom to this book, as I know your insights will inspire many other midwives too.

What can you learn from Franka's journey in leadership?

LEADING WITH COMPASSION

Compassionate leadership in healthcare has become established as a route towards cultivating wisdom, humanity, presence and high quality in healthcare services. Compassionate leadership is particularly aligned with the approaches we touch on within this book. Broadly speaking, compassionate leadership involves attending to, understanding, empathising with and helping those we lead (West 2021).

When exploring what shows compassion in healthcare (Clyne et al. 2018), participants described how 'leaders must role model positive behaviours and values' and how 'compassion is a key component of leadership'. Ultimately, 'leadership and the right culture is essential' in the demonstration of workplace compassion. This research also contributed to the development of NHS England's and NHS Improvement's Resource pack to support workplace compassion and support guide towards commissioning for workplace compassion (see resources section for full web addresses).

Compassionate leaders are emotionally in touch with others in their workplace. According to Ashkanasy and Humphrey (2011), emotion operates throughout organisations at five different levels. These broadly resonate as follows:

Level one: The individual behaviours and emotional states and reactions of people on a day-to-day basis

Level two: Different attitudes and learnt behaviour of staff including different levels of emotional intelligence

Level three: The perception and communication of emotions between staff

Level four: Group dynamics within teams including leadership influence, performance and behaviour

Level five: The emotional climate of an organisation linked to its performance

As a leader, it will be important for you to manage and understand emotion in each of these levels. Emotional intelligence is a term used to describe one's capacity to identify, assess and regulate their emotions, as well as the emotions of individuals and of groups in the organisation, of which there are five interrelated aspects (Goleman 1996, pp. 49–50):

1. Self-awareness (e.g. recognition of your own values, goals, strengths and weaknesses and their impact upon others)
2. Motivation/passion (e.g. ability to stimulate people to willingly work towards goals)
3. Empathy (e.g. ability to understand and connect with other people's emotions through similar experiences)
4. Social skills (e.g. your abilities to understand, influence and manage people)
5. Self-regulation/management (e.g. ability to adapt to changing circumstances).

In leading compassionately, you will also need to build trust between you and your followers. If you as a leader believe that your followers are truthful, they are indeed more likely to be (Goman 2020). Brower et al. (2017) usefully set out four ways in which trust can be fostered:

1. Let trust create trust (e.g. demonstrate that you trust your followers [for example, through delegation] and they will reciprocate).
2. Share information to avoid distrust in withholding it
3. Balance risk aversion and communication
4. Care for your followers (e.g. through supporting future development)

Below is a useful reflection suggested by Delizonna (2017) to aid you in maintaining compassion and speaking 'human to human' called 'Just Like Me,' which asks you to consider in situations of conflict that:

- This person has beliefs, perspectives and opinions, just like me.
- This person has hopes, anxieties and vulnerabilities, just like me.
- This person has friends, family and perhaps children who love them, just like me.
- This person wants to feel respected, appreciated and competent, just like me.
- This person wishes for peace, joy and happiness, just like me.

The Founding Director of Midwife-led Community Transformation (MILCOT), Harriet Nayiga from Uganda, shared her thoughts with us about leading change with compassion for her team and the surrounding community:

'MILCOT is a community-based organisation that brings midwifery services out of labour ward and makes them closer to the community through preventive initiatives rather than responding to complications. MILCOT aims at bridging the gap between midwives and the community through the provision of sexual reproductive health rights, survival skills and psychological support to marginalised adolescents and young adults focusing on prevention of teenage and unplanned pregnancies.

Since 2017 when I decided to do charity, life has never been easy, surviving and thriving has been by the grace of God, it's about sacrifice and sharing the little that I have with those who are in most need. My survival story began from offering my house to serve as organisation's office to sometimes foregoing lunch to buy internet to facilitate work.

My community work is done under meagre resources to ensure that marginalised adolescents and young adults survive and thrive with safe livelihood. I and my team work on a volunteer basis in reaching out to marginalised adolescents and young adults with sexual reproductive health information and services. The girls also come to the centre for their vocational skilling classes where they interact with fellows, get psychosocial support and also get lunch which is unusual in their homes.

(continued)

(continued)

Majority of the girls depend on hand to mouth by doing petty jobs like washing clothes in homesteads to get what to eat. I got so worried when the pandemic came, the girls could not move to carry out their work and it was tough to get a meal. In addition to the relief fund that supported them with food, sanitary pads and other items, I used to call them on the phone for counselling. During the second wave of COVID-19, MIL-COT did not receive a relief fund, the girls came to office one day to ask for something to eat and feed their babies. I portioned the little food which I had stocked for myself, and I gave them to go and cook. These were tough moments that I would not wish to see again.

On the other hand, midwives in the community were afraid of the devastating situation of COVID-19 and they needed psychosocial support. Through the Nursing Now Challenge project, I and my team empowered them with resilience skills to go through these tough times and developed their leadership skills. My means of surviving and thriving has been through extending compassion to my team and the people around me and I have never lost hope because this is my purpose, I have surrounded myself with mentors, partners and people who encourage and support me. Through endless efforts in mobilising resources, partners have stood with us to serve the community. I would have no reasons to smile amidst this pool of challenges but the impact that my work has made gives me a smile and gives me endless strength and hope.

Midwifery is a calling where people see us as their saviours and yet working under unfavourable conditions, the only way to survive and thrive is by taking up our position, advocating for what we need so that we effectively help women and children. "When you realize that you are weak but stronger than some, you gain strength through helping those who are weak. We are strong together"'

Harriet Nayiga – Founding Director of Midwife-led Community Transformation (MILCOT)

LIFTING OTHERS UP AS YOU CLIMB

In effectively leading teams and creating psychological safety, you will be able to lift up colleagues as you climb (See Chapter 5). In creating psychological safety in your own team, you will see higher levels of engagement, increased motivation to tackle difficult problems, more learning and development opportunities and better performance. Successful teams will have universal needs such as respect, competence, social status and autonomy. In forging your own successful team of psychologically safe colleagues, try replicating the following steps outlined by Delizonna (2017):

1. **Approach conflict as a collaborator, not an adversary**: Instead ask, how might we achieve a mutually desirable outcome?
2. **Speak human to human:** Even in the most provocative of situations, it is important to remember that colleagues are just like you (consider the 'just like you' reflection outlined in Section 8.5).

3. **Anticipate reactions and plan countermoves:** In this, consider how your message will be heard and prepare for likely reactions. In this, you can avoid your messages being heard as a personal attack on the ego and instead ensure that your message is communicated with compassion.

4. **Replace blame with curiosity:** Blame can lead to defensiveness which in turn leads to disengagement. Instead, try to adopt a learning mindset in terms of what went wrong.

5. **Ask for feedback on delivery:** When delivering bad news, this essentially disarms those ready to oppose you, and role models' fallibility to increase trust.

6. **Measure psychological safety:** In cultivating this, actively ask how psychologically safe the team feel and what could enhance their feeling of safety. An example question might be: 'How confident are you that you won't receive retaliation or criticism if you admit an error or make a mistake?'

Throughout our professional lives, we will always do better when we see the best rather than the worst in each other. So, when we see a colleague fall, let us lift them up rather than tear them down. Moreover, there is really no need to tell the world they fell in the first place.

> *To me, a leader is someone who holds her- or himself accountable for finding potential in people and processes.*
>
> – Brené Brown

IN CONVERSATION (SALLY AND KAREN EXPLORE PERSONAL INSIGHTS ON LEADERSHIP)

KM   Is there someone in your career that you hold up as an example of a great leader? What did they do that makes you feel that way?

SP   This is easy – Janet Fyle, policy officer for the RCM has always been someone I have looked up to. She saw my potential a few years ago now and invested solidly in helping me realise it. Having someone celebrate and value me in that way made me step up my game. I had to live up to what they saw in me. I watch Janet lead others in doing the same and I am in awe of her. Janet's legacy will undoubtedly live on through every midwife who has had the honour of ever being in her presence.

KM   Having that role model and mentor to show you the way is so valuable for us to achieve our potential. They don't even have to be in a formal mentoring or leadership role, or even in your own workplace. Some of the most valuable mentoring and leadership role modelling for me have come through my informal network. Having those more informal mentors can help us see perhaps when our own workplace isn't working for us or to open new opportunities that we hadn't considered. So, do you think that anyone can lead? Or are there special skills that people need to develop first?

SP   I think there are certainly people who are born with innate leadership skills, though surely developing any leadership skills further is always a bonus! People do seem to gravitate towards me as a leader, and I have been fortunate enough to have many professional development opportunities and complete many programmes and qualifications in leadership. I hope this investment in myself has made me a better leader.

KM   I think all the courses and executive development programmes that are available highlight that leadership is definitely a learnable skill. From your time on these programmes what have you learnt about your own leadership practice?

SP   I have certainly learnt to navigate and use certain organisational values and strategies to my advantage. However, I am constantly aware of the barriers I face as a cisgender woman in taking advantage of high-level leadership opportunities. Nevertheless, I do sometimes wonder whether I may achieve a greater impact leading on the projects I care about without the constraints of a high-level position in leadership.

KM   You can definitely lead without a 'leadership' title, and I think each of us can lead in our own way. Leadership with a little 'l'. It's all about bringing people with you and having something that others want to follow. Was there anything on the programmes that surprised you and made you want to include in your own leadership practice or felt that midwifery would benefit from?

SP   I think in midwifery, and healthcare in general we are always having to navigate complex changes. What I valued most was the skills I learnt in leading through change. Whilst change is never easy, I expect midwifery is on the cusp of having to be reimagined if the profession is to thrive and keep pace in the everchanging context of reproduction.

KM   It is an interesting time and one thing we can all be certain of is change. It is all around us all the time. How we can either lead others or be led through the uncertainty of a change process is integral to what the outcome of the change looks like. Trust and communication are two important aspects in the management literature for leading others and key to positive working relationships during the change process so are there any small things you do every day that help to build positive relationships with others or a sense of community?

SP   The specific coaching behaviours I offer include authentic role modelling, praise and encouragement. I also focus on the building of trust and mutual respect. It's so important to lift others up as you climb. I guess that's part of the reason for wanting to write this book. Yet I also give a lot of time acting as a PhD supervisor and as a coach/mentor to midwives and nurses through various avenues. This gives me a great sense of well-being and community within the profession. After all, midwifery leaders build on the legacy we leave.

Activity – Leadership on Improvement Project

In your own sphere of practice, identify a problem that needs fixing in practice. Start small. (you can always go big later!) For example, is there a better way to manage the shift rota? A better way to transport people between departments or keep hygiene standards high? Architect a solution to a small problem you see in your own area in partnership with colleagues. This is the first step of a Plan, Do, Check, Act (PDCA) Cycle. This may seem like a simple cycle, but it can be highly effective in leading change. As you progress through the steps, think about how you are bringing people with you (leading) on your journey. What leadership skills will you build on to succeed in your quest? Continue to follow these steps of the cycle as follows:

Plan: Identify a problem in need of resolve in practice. Be sure to look at the root causes of this problem and set goals to overcome it.

Do: Once you have decided on a course of action in partnership with colleagues, lead on exploring and testing the different ways you might achieve your goals together.

Check: Review progress towards your goals regularly. Adjust your approaches accordingly, whilst considering any potential consequences.

Act: Lead on the implementation of what works best. You will need to continue to refine your solutions, by returning to the beginning of the cycle.

CHAPTER 9

Turning Visions into Practice

INTRO TO CHAPTER

Many, but not all, of the issues and challenges within this book have the potential to be modified through self-development and problem-solving. That said, it is not our intention to minimise any of the acutely real, structural and systemic issues within midwifery today, and much discussion of how these could be overcome has been presented by other authors (Homer et al. 2014). Our aim is to arm current and future midwives with the tools and resources to successfully navigate their careers and provide the best perinatal care for as long as possible. When working in such a multi-faceted and interconnected system such as healthcare often the only elements under our control are within us: our thoughts, actions and interactions. Through working individually on those things under our control we can effect a cultural change in midwifery from the ground up and send a ripple effect outwards across our organisations.

In this chapter, we provide an evidence-based framework for making a meaningful change within our control that can send ripples out across our teams, organisations and the profession. If each midwife who reads this book vows to make one small change, these can add up to one huge change with the potential to shift the profession in a different direction. The aim of this chapter is to encourage you to be the change you want to see.

GOAL SETTING

Goal setting has been used within coaching for decades in order to drive performance and motivation across a range of disciplines including sport, business, education, life coaching and health behaviours. Traditionally, goal setting has focused on concrete

Surviving and Thriving in Midwifery, First Edition. Sally Pezaro and Karen Maher.
© 2025 John Wiley & Sons Ltd. Published 2025 by John Wiley & Sons Ltd.

objective measures of performance as they are easy to quantify and therefore know whether they have been achieved. Setting specific and challenging, but achievable goals leads to better performance than setting vague goals or 'doing your best'. Using tools such as SMART (specific, measurable, achievable, realistic, time-bound) goals to create goal statements provides a foundation from which to access performance measures.

- **S**pecific (simple/significant)
- **M**easurable (meaningful/motivating)
- **A**chievable (attainable/agreed upon)
- **R**ealistic (reasonable/resourced)
- **T**ime-bound (time/cost limited)

Locke and Latham are key researchers in the field of goal setting and have identified different factors that can influence the success, or otherwise of your goal attempts. Spending time reflecting on these when setting goals can help identify potential barriers and blocks to goal success. Some are internal to us, such as how much we value the goal or the outcome, the amount of effort we put into working on the goal and our beliefs about how well we can perform the goal. Others are related to the goal itself, such as how complex it is, whether it is specific and challenging, whether there are opportunities for feedback.

Taking a solely objective quantitative approach to goal setting risks goal setting becoming a cold and remote activity with the emphasis on the outcome more than the person or the process. It is also limited in the ability to develop 'soft skills' or growth goals that are often intangible and difficult to objectively measure. Personal and/or professional growth goals are linked to higher levels of well-being through being a catalyst for positive change (Travers et al. 2014) and if the growth goal you choose to work on is energising and holds your focus, effort and persistence then your personal and/or professional outcomes should improve. When focusing on growth goals a vital part of the process is reflection: at the start of the process in order to identify a suitable goal, during the goal attempt to identify whether any modifications are needed, and then after the goal attempt to identify what worked and plan for future attempts. Thus, the process of goal setting becomes cyclical where there is continuous refinement and personal growth. Travers and colleagues developed a five-stage cycle of reflective goal setting to support soft skill development and growth goals with writing things down as you go through the cycle as a key element to successful outcomes in Figure 9.1 outlined below. Writing provides a vehicle for awareness of things that are important to attend to, structure and understand thoughts and emotions, leaving a record available for review and insight later which can all strengthen the goal attainment process. Travers suggests keeping a diary with regular entries (no fewer than three times a week) right from the point at which you are thinking of working on a goal. Early entries can help enhance self-awareness and refine your goal statement with later entries becoming more reflective on the goal attempts themselves.

If you have an area of personal or professional development you wish to work on, the following section will guide you through how to apply the reflective goal setting cycle to your goals. The first step is to create a diary that can be handwritten or digital,

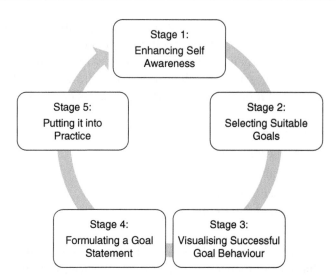

FIGURE 9.1   Reflective goal setting cycle. *Source*: Reproduced from Travers, 2022 / with permission of Springer Nature.

however the benefits of having a handwritten diary are that it is a permanent record that cannot be easily edited. Your diary then becomes the place where you record your thoughts and reflections on each of the stages as you go through the cycle.

Stage 1: Enhancing self-awareness – the purpose of this part of the process is to identify a suitable goal for personal development. This may be easy because there has been something hanging around for a long time that you have felt would be beneficial to work on for either your career or personal development, or it could be more challenging if you are not clear about the challenges you face or areas you would like to grow. The key in this stage is using as many points of reference as possible to gain insight and increase self-awareness.

- Identify self-awareness activities in which you could engage using your diary as a store for your responses. What do personality tests tell you about how you approach problems at work? Can stress questionnaires guide your understanding of how you are coping with challenges? What can you understand about your communication style, leadership style, empathy/emotional intelligence and how might that influence the areas you wish to work on?
- Gather and evaluate feedback from multiple sources such as annual appraisals, midwifery placement logs from training, even school/university reports. Are there common areas that cut across all your different types of feedback? Is there one area of feedback that has the potential for a growth goal that could have a big impact on your life/career?
- Use your diary to reflect on personal life experiences and behaviour patterns. What can you understand about how you have dealt with critical incidents in your work or more generally? Are there common patterns of behaviour that are helpful/unhelpful? How do others react to you? Are your behaviours consistent across groups of people or do you behave differently when with those in your care, colleagues, your social group? Why might that be?

- Uncover and understand what matters to you – your values (see Chapter 2). What drives you in life and your career? What values do you choose to live your life by? What opportunities do you get to express these at work/in life?
- Consider what those close to you need from you. What do the different people in your life (family, colleagues, maternity service users) need in terms of your behaviours and actions? How do those needs conjoin/conflict?

Stage 2: Selecting suitable goals – Once you have gone through the process of in-depth self-awareness the next stage is to start to develop a goal focus. At this stage this can be quite broad using the reflection process to gradually refine the growth goal area. Use your diary to reflect on:

- Identifying a specific but challenging goal area, for example, you may identify through your self-awareness activities that you want to develop your assertiveness in order to manage your personal boundaries or use healthier coping mechanisms when under pressure.
- Consider scenarios where you could benefit from an improvement. This could be at work engaging with those in your care and/or colleagues, or outside of work with family or other people close to you. The more specific the scenario the more concrete your final goal statement will be.
- Understand what your current behaviour looks like in relation to this goal. For example, what do you currently do when someone violates a boundary such as talking over you in front of someone you are supporting through their pregnancy or birth experience or in a team meeting? What actions do you take when you feel under pressure?
- Feedback from significant others about your potential goal area. Do they think it would be a good idea to work on? Can they see the benefits? Are they open to supporting you?

Stage 3: Visualise successful goal behaviours – Here the idea is to really understand what success looks like through visualising what it would look like to perform the ideal behaviour. By exploring the gap between current and ideal behaviours can help to identify ways to measure your outcomes or success. Sometimes this might involve a distinct measurement tool (stress scale, for example) but it may also be through your personal reflections such as the times you were able to assert your boundaries. Use your diary to reflect on:

- The specific behaviours and outcomes you want to see when you are successful. What actions will you be taking when carrying out the goal successfully? What will others see when you are successful? How will it feel when you are carrying out your goal?
- Any role models or past behaviour or good practice. Who performs this goal in a way that you would like to? Have you successfully carried out this goal in the past? If so, what were the conditions around that successful attempt? Are there any examples of good practice in this goal (could be written down in terms of policy or visual guides or evidence from literature) that exist?

- Compare your ideal with your current behaviour. How far is the gap between them? What do you need to do to move from current behaviour to the ideal? Do you need to break the gap down into smaller steps to make the final goal more achievable?

Stage 4: Formulate a goal statement – When formulating your goal statement, it needs to provide an overview of the goal behaviour, desired goal outcome, the techniques to be used to achieve the goal and the ways in which you will measure progress and success. The more clearly these are articulated the greater the level of your commitment towards the goal. Use your diary to outline your goal statement:

- State the specific goal action e.g. *to enhance*
- Identify a specific performance area e.g. *assertiveness*
- Identify specific scenarios related to your goal action e.g. *in team meetings/ shift handover*
- Select specific techniques and approaches to use e.g. *by saying no when I am unable to take on extra work/using I statements when putting my point across*
- Identify measurements or standards e.g. *my own reflections on feeling a greater sense of control/or lower stress scores*
- Give a timeframe or deadline e.g. *by my appraisal*

Stage 5: Putting it into practice – Find opportunities to put your goal actions into practice and then use your diary to reflect on how it went. Explore how it felt, what went well, what could be improved. As you are keeping a record of your goal attempts, these reflections can be used as a measure of success and growth towards your ideal. These reflections should be used to adjust your goal statement as and when necessary. For example, it may be that the techniques you decided to use did not work or were not right for you and therefore you can try a different one or you may wish to review the measurement criteria to ensure it is right for the desired outcome that you have.

As this is a reflective goal setting cycle, once you have successfully completed the goal and your ideal behaviour is now your current behaviour, you can start the process again and set a new goal so that self-development becomes a continuous process.

Whilst it is all very well and exciting to set your goals, it will also be crucial to work towards achieving them too. In the following section, we will explore how you can work towards achieving the goals you set and how those actions may or may not fit into wider change within the midwifery context.

BE THE CHANGE YOU WANT TO SEE

Why do we want and need to change?

If you want to lead change, it will be important to understand change in the context of leadership (e.g. see Godbole 2017) and why change might be resisted in your particular context. Kotter and Schlesinger (1989) have identified four well-established reasons why people may resist change. Do you recognise any of them in yourself or in others?

1. **Parochial self-interest:** Essentially, individuals worry that the change will cause them to lose something (e.g. status or power). Self-interest may develop as one gets a sense that the change is perceived to be in misalignment with what one believes is in their best interests.

2. **Misunderstanding and lack of trust:** Uncertainty during the process of change can lead to misunderstandings and subsequent distrust. This is where strong communication is needed, particularly where followers believe the reward to be less than the costs involved in embracing the change.

3. **Different assessments:** Quite simply, others may not agree with the proposed changes and assess them differently. In this sense, they may not see it as being beneficial and resist, particularly where people are in possession of different information.

4. **Low tolerance for change:** The process of change may cause stress and anxiety for some, particularly if they do not feel well able to adapt or fear that they will not have the skills and knowledge required once the proposed changes are implemented. In such cases, one might resist change, even if they agree with it in principle.

So, once you understand how yourself and the people around you may resist change, it will be important for you to develop strategies in relation to how you will overcome these and achieve the changes you want to see in the midwifery world. In this task, Kotter and Schlesinger (1989) once again suggest six useful strategies for dealing with resistance to change:

1. **Education and communication:** As many of the reasons for resistance relate to crossed wires in communication and access to different sources of information during the processes of change, it makes sense to counter these elements with strong communication strategies and education throughout the change process. In communicating the reasons for change effectively, followers may be better able to understand why the change is needed. Invest time and effort to build relationships of trust where information can be shared with honesty and openness to avoid the miscommunications and misinterpretations that can lead to resistance.

2. **Participation and involvement:** Whilst it may not be feasible in cases requiring urgency, participation and involvement in the change as it unfolds may enable followers to become invested in the change once committed.

3. **Facilitation and support:** In order to ensure a smoother transition through change, it is useful to consider what followers may need in terms of support (e.g. training, mentoring, counselling). Taking time in getting this right may be useful in helping people adjust, particularly where people are anxious or stressed in relation to the change.

4. **Negotiation and agreement:** If an individual or group has significant power in resisting proposed changes, there may be value in bargaining with them to either change or leave. This may be particularly useful where a restructuring of teams or processes is required.

5. **Manipulation and co-optation:** Whilst manipulation may seem unethical, sometimes the use of selective information may be beneficial in cases where there is seemingly no other way forward in overcoming resistance. Co-optation may also be useful in getting the support of someone who may otherwise be resistant to the change and 'onboarding' them in the change efforts.

6. **Explicit and implicit coercion:** This is a risky strategy as people are bound to strongly resist enforced change. Yet the ultimatum of either job loss or promotion, for example, may be the only options leaders of change are left with.

Ultimately, the key to dealing with supporters of change is to work out how to mobilise them into action and commit to achieving a shared new goal. In this task, you may usefully mix enthusiastic and motivating supporters with resisters, the latter of whom either need to be engaged or neutralised. In this, you will need to ascertain how much power the resister holds in thwarting the change, and whether their resistance is due to either inertia (e.g. they just like the status quo and may need waking up to new ways of doing and being) or passive (e.g. they do not like change but may open to persuasions or incentives to change). Once you make these assessments, you can then go about managing the changes you want to see in the world. In this, it will be useful to demonstrate and celebrate quick wins and generate a supportive and compelling narrative or story of the change as it takes place. Before any change takes place, openness, readiness and commitment to the change will be key in ensuring success.

IN CONVERSATION (SALLY AND KAREN'S FINAL REFLECTIONS)

KB We've come to the end of the book. How have you found the process of writing it and our conversations for each chapter?

SP I am grateful for all of the times we have the opportunity to work and chat together. I have also been humbled by the number of stories we have been able to include from other midwives around the world to support the ideas and tools we had the vision to share.

KB Absolutely, I am so grateful to every single midwife who has shared their story, and it adds a real richness to the book. What do you hope other midwives will take away from reading the book?

SP The profession needs every midwife to thrive. This is what I try to remember when it feels like the world is trying to drag me down. I hope other midwives can draw strength and learn from the experiences I have shared here, as well as from those shared by others. I want midwives to thrive, and I see potential everywhere I look. Yet sometimes it feels as if midwives are waiting for permission. Now is our time!

KB   It is an interesting time in midwifery across the world. What do you hope for the future of midwifery, both in the United Kingdom where you are based, but also globally where you have already reached so many other colleagues through your work?

SP   If midwives are to assist in reaching the United Nations Sustainable Development Goals, particularly with regard to equality, which will ultimately lead to greater health and well-being worldwide, then the midwifery profession will require somewhat of a contemporary reimagining. Midwifery needs to move towards being inclusive of all people who birth (not just cisgender women) and be proactive (rather than reactive) in supporting and retaining staff in a profession that is attractive and psychologically safe to join in the first place. Historical and reflective narratives of midwifery may be a useful way to instantiate and ground the contemporary and future identity of midwifery as we go towards the middle of the twenty-first century and beyond. The best is yet to come!

We both thank you for investing your time and yourselves in reading this book. We hope it has enriched you and that you will draw back to it throughout your career in midwifery. We would be keen to know how this book is being used to make a change in the world. Please do get in touch or find us on social media to share your impact and success stories!

– Dr Sally Pezaro and Dr Karen Maher

Recommended Resources and Links to Organisations

CHAPTER 1

Dahlen, H.G., K.-H, B., and S, V. (2020). *Birthing Outside the System: The Canary in the Coal Mine*. Routledge.

Feeley, C. 'Practising Outside of the Box, whilst within the System': A Feminist Narrative Inquiry of NHS Midwives Supporting and Facilitating Women's Alternative Physiological Birthing Choices. Doctoral Dissertation, University of Central Lancashire, 2019.

Feeley, C. (2022). The ASSET model: what midwives need to support alternative physiological births (outwith guidelines). *The Practising Midwife* 25 (2): 26–30.

Sarah W. (2021). In Your Own Time: How Western Medicine Controls the Start of Labour and why this Needs to Stop, Birthmoon Creations.

CHAPTER 2

Living Life to the Full – Free Cognitive Behavioural Therapy Resources to Work Through at Your Own Pace. https://llttf.com

Kabat-Zinn, J. (2013). *Full Catastrophe Living; How to Cope with Stress, Pain and Illness Using Mindfulness Mediation*. London: Piatkus.

Williams, M. and Penman, D. (2011). *Mindfulness: A Practical Guide for Finding Peace in a Frantic World*. London: Piatkus.

CHAPTER 3

Health and Safety Executive Stress Tools and Templates. www.hse.gov.uk/stress/standards/downloads.htm

CHAPTER 4

For support with substance use further information, guidance and resources can be found via Alcoholics Anonymous and Narcotics Anonymous with country specific resources available.

Surviving and Thriving in Midwifery, First Edition. Sally Pezaro and Karen Maher.
© 2025 John Wiley & Sons Ltd. Published 2025 by John Wiley & Sons Ltd.

Drink Calculator. `https://alcoholchange.org.uk/alcohol-facts/interactive-tools/unit-calculator`

CHAPTER 5

Royal College of Obstetricians and Gynecologists (RCOG's). Workplace Behaviour Toolkit. `www.rcog.org.uk/careers-and-training/starting-your-og-career/workforce/improving-workplace-behaviours/workplace-behaviour-toolkit`

Civility Toolkit: Resources to Empower Healthcare Leaders to Identify, Intervene, and Prevent Workplace Bullying. Passionate About Creating Environments of Respect and Civilities. `http://stopbullyingtoolkit.org`

Healthy Workforce Institute. `https://healthyworkforceinstitute.com/resources`

Resources for employer: workplace bullying. American Psychological Association Center for Organizational Excellence. `https://www.apaexcellence.org/resources/special-topics/workplace-bullying`

#Saynotobullyinginmidwifery report: `www.midwifery.org.uk/our-shop/saynotobullyinginmidwifery-report`

Stop Bullying on the Spot. `www.stopbullying.gov`

Violence, Incivility, & Bullying. American Nurses Association. `https://www.nursingworld.org/practice-policy/work-environment/violence-incivility-bullying`

A Manifesto for Change: Prioritise Nurses, Midwives and Paramedics' Psychological Health to Strengthen the NHS Culture. `www.surrey.ac.uk/news/manifesto-change-prioritise-nurses-midwives-and-paramedics-psychological-health-strengthen-nhs`

The Joint Commission's Sentinel Event Alert Outlining the Ways in Which Health Care Leaders Should Address Workplace Bullying: `https://www.jointcommission.org/resources/patient-safety-topics/sentinel-event/sentinel-event-alert-newsletters/sentinel-event-alert-issue-40-behaviors-that-undermine-a-culture-of-safety`

CHAPTER 6

Edmondson, A.C. (2018). *The Fearless Organization: Creating Psychological Safety in the Workplace for Learning, Innovation, and Growth*. Wiley.

CHAPTER 7

Murray, R. and Moore, S. (2006). *The Handbook of Academic Writing: A Fresh Approach*. Maidenhead: Open University Press.

CHAPTER 8

Florence Nightingale Foundation Leadership Programmes. `https://florence-nightingale-foundation.org.uk/academy/leadership-development/leadership-programmes`

NHS Resource Pack to Support Workplace Compassion. `https://www.england.nhs.uk/wp-content/uploads/2018/10/resource-pack-to-support-workplace-compassion-march-2020.pdf`

NHS England Support Guide for Commissioning for Workplace Compassion. `https://www.england.nhs.uk/wp-content/uploads/2018/10/towards-commissioning-for-workplace-compassion-a-support-guide-v2.pdf`

CHAPTER 9

Travers, C.J. (2022). *Reflective Goal Setting: An Applied Approach to Personal and Leadership Development*. Palgrave Macmillan.

Appendix

List of Values

Acceptance	Co-operation	Focus	Insightful	Professionalism	Status
Accomplishment	Creativity	Fortitude	Inspiring	Purpose	Strength
Accountability	Credibility	Freedom	Integrity	Quality	Success
Accuracy	Curiosity	Friendship	Intelligence	Reason	Support
Achievement	Decisive	Fun	Joy	Recognition	Sustainability
Adaptability	Dedication	Generosity	Justice	Reflective	Teamwork
Altruism	Dependability	Giving	Kindness	Respect	Temperance
Ambition	Development	Grace	Leadership	Responsibility	Thankful
Assertiveness	Dignity	Gratitude	Learning	Rigour	Thorough
Balance	Discipline	Growth	Love	Risk	Thoughtful
Beauty	Discovery	Happiness	Loyalty	Satisfaction	Tolerance
Boldness	Effectiveness	Hard work	Mastery	Security	Toughness
Bravery	Efficiency	Harmony	Openness	Selfless	Traditional
Calm	Empathy	Health	Optimism	Sensitivity	Tranquillity
Candor	Empowerment	Honesty	Organisation	Serenity	Trust
Capable	Enthusiasm	Hope	Originality	Simplicity	Truth
Certainty	Equality	Humility	Passion	Sincerity	Understanding
Challenge	Ethical	Humour	Patience	Skill	Unity
Charity	Experience	Imagination	Peace	Solitude	Vigour
Commitment	Fairness	Independence	Persistence	Spirituality	Vision
Community	Family	Individuality	Playfulness	Spontaneous	Wealth
Compassion	Fearless	Innovation	Power	Stability	Wisdom

Surviving and Thriving in Midwifery, First Edition. Sally Pezaro and Karen Maher.
© 2025 John Wiley & Sons Ltd. Published 2025 by John Wiley & Sons Ltd.

References

Altman, D.G. and Simera, I. (2014). Using reporting guidelines effectively to ensure good reporting of health research. In: *Guidelines for Reporting Health Research: A User's Manual* (ed. D. Moher, D.G. Altman, K.F. Schulz, et al.), 32–40. Wiley https://doi.org/10.1002/9781118715598.ch4.

Anderson, J.E. and Watt, A.J. (2020). Using safety-II and resilient healthcare principles to learn from never events. *International Journal for Quality in Health Care* 32(3): 196–203. https://doi.org/10.1093/intqhc/mzaa009.

Anisman, H. (2014). *An Introduction to Stress and Health*. SAGE Publications, Inc.

Anzaldua, A. and Halpern, J. (2021). Can clinical empathy survive? Distress, burnout, and malignant duty in the age of Covid-19. *Hastings Center Report* 51(1): 22–27. https://doi.org/10.1002/hast.1216.

Appelbaum, E., Bailey, T., Berg, P., and Kalleberg, A. (2000). *Manufacturing Advantage: Why High-Performance Work Systems Pay Off*. Cornell University Press.

Arena, M.J. and Uhl-Bien, M. (2016). Complexity leadership theory: shifting from human capital to social capital. *The Leadership Quarterly* 39(2): 631–650. https://doi.org/10.1016/j.leaqua.2009.04.007.

Ashakanasy, N.M. and Humphrey, R.H. (2011). A multi-level view of leadership and emotion: leading with emotional labor. In: *The SAGE Handbook of Leadership*, 365–379. SAGE Publications, Inc.

Avolio, B.J. and Gardner, W.L. (2005). Authentic leadership development: getting to the root of positive forms of leadership. *The Leadership Quarterly* 16(3): 315–338. https://doi.org/10.1016/j.leaqua.2005.03.001.

Baldisseri, M.R. (2007). Impaired healthcare professional. *Critical Care Medicine* 35 (2 SUPPL): https://doi.org/10.1097/01.CCM.0000252918.87746.96.

Bass, B.M. (1985). *Leadership and Performance Beyond Expectations*. Free Press.

Bass, B.M. (1997). Does the transactional-transformational leadership paradigm transcend organizational and national boundaries? *American Psychologist*, 52(2), 130-139.

Bass, B.M. and Yammarino, F.J. (1991). Congruence of self and others' leadership ratings of naval officers for understanding successful performance. *Applied Psychology* 40(4): 437–454.

Bekhruz, B. (2022). The difference between a leader and a boss in management. *Galaxy International Interdisciplinary Research Journal* 10(2): 135–137.

Surviving and Thriving in Midwifery, First Edition. Sally Pezaro and Karen Maher.
© 2025 John Wiley & Sons Ltd. Published 2025 by John Wiley & Sons Ltd.

Bernstein, S.L., Kelechi, T.J., Catchpole, K., and Nemeth, L.S. (2021). Prevention of failure to rescue in obstetric patients: a realist review. *Worldviews on Evidence-Based Nursing* 18(6): 352–360. https://doi.org/10.1111/wvn.12531.

Boyer, E.L. (1990). *Scholarship Reconsidered: Priorities of the Professoriate*. Carnegie Foundation for the Advancement of Teaching.

Brand, A., Allen, L., Altman, M. et al. (2015). Beyond authorship: attribution, contribution, collaboration, and credit. *Learned Publishing* 28(2): 151–155. https://doi.org/10.1087/20150211.

Bridgewater St Mary's Parish Records (1682). *Baptisms 1682-1714; Marriages 1682-1714; Burials 1682-1714*. Somerset Records Office.

Brower, H.H., Lester, S.W., and Korsgaard, M.A. (2017). Want your employees to trust you? Show you trust them. *Harvard Business Review* 47: 81–89.

Brown, B. (2006). Shame resilience theory: a grounded theory study on women and shame. *Families in Society: The Journal of Contemporary Social Services* 87(1): 43–52. https://doi.org/10.1606/1044-3894.3483.

Burns, J.M. (1978). *Leadership*. Harper and Row.

Capaldi, C.A., Passmore, H.-A., Nisbet, E.K. et al. (2015). Flourishing in nature: a review of the benefits of connecting with nature and its application as a wellbeing intervention. *International Journal of Wellbeing* 5(4): 1–16.

Capper, T.S., Muurlink, O.T., and Williamson, M.J. (2021). The parents are watching: midwifery students' perceptions of how workplace bullying impacts mothers and babies. *Midwifery* 103: 103144. https://doi.org/10.1016/j.midw.2021.103144.

Capper, T., Ferguson, B., and Muurlink, O. (2024). Health professionals' experiences of whistleblowing in maternal and newborn healthcare settings: a scoping review and thematic analysis. *Women and Birth* 101593. https://doi.org/10.1016/j.wombi.2024.101593.

Chadwick, R.J. (2022). Visceral acts: gestationality as feminist figuaration. *Signs: Journal of Women in Culture and Society* 48(1): 229–255.

Chitongo, S., Pezaro, S., Fyle, J. et al. (2022). Midwives' insights in relation to the common barriers in providing effective perinatal care to women from ethnic minority groups with 'high risk' pregnancies: a qualitative study. *Women and Birth* 35(2): 152–159. https://doi.org/10.1016/j.wombi.2021.05.005.

Civial Aviation Authority (2016). Situational awareness. In: *Flight Crew Human Factors Handbook*. Civil Aviation Authority.

Clyne, W., Pezaro, S., Deeny, K., and Kneafsey, R. (2018). Using social media to generate and collect primary data: the #ShowsWorkplaceCompassion twitter research campaign. *JMIR Public Health and Surveillance* 4(2): e41. https://doi.org/10.2196/publichealth.7686.

Cody, L.F. (2005). *Birthing the Nation: Sex, Science, and the Conception of Eighteenth-century Britons*. Oxford University Press.

Collins, J.C. and Porras, J.T. (1991). Organisational vision and visioning organisations. *California Management Review* 34(1): 30–52.

Cooley, C. (1902). Looking glass self. In: *The Production of Reality: Essays and Readings on Social Interaction*, vol. 6, 126–128. Sage.

Craig, N. and Snook, S.A. (2014). From purpose to impact. *Harvard Business Review* 92(5): 104–111.

Davis, D.E., Ho, M.Y., Griffin, B.J. et al. (2015). Forgiving the self and physical and mental health correlates: a meta-analytic review. *Journal of Counseling Psychology* 62(2): 329–335. https://doi.org/10.1037/cou0000063.

Delizonna, L. (2017). High-performing teams need psychological safety. Here's how to create it. *Harvard Business Review* 8: 1–5.

d'Ettorre, G., Ceccarelli, G., Santinelli, L. et al. (2021). Post-traumatic stress symptoms in healthcare workers dealing with the COVID-19 pandemic: a systematic review. *International Journal of Environmental Research and Public Health* 18(2): 601. https://doi.org/10.3390/ijerph18020601.

Dollard, M.F. and Bakker, A.B. (2010). Psychosocial safety climate as a precursor to conducive work environments, psychological health problems, and employee engagement. *Journal of Occupational and Organizational Psychology* 83(3): 579–599. https://doi.org/10.1348/096317909X470690.

Drucker, P.F. (1967). The effective decision. In: *Harvard Business Review on Decision Making*, 1–8. Harvard Business School Publishing.

Edmondson, A. (1996). Learning from mistakes is easier said than done: group and organsiational influences on the detection and correction of human error. *The Journal of Applied Behavioral Science* 35: 5–32.

Edmondson, A. (1999). Psychological safety and learning behavior in work teams. *Administrative Science Quarterly* 44(2): 350–383. https://doi.org/10.2307/2666999.

Edmondson, A.C. (2011). Strategies for learning from failure. *Harvard Business Review* 89(4): 48–55.

Ellis, A. and Ellis, D.J. (2019). *Rational Emotive Behaviour Therapy*, 2e. American Psychological Association.

Enright, R.D. and Fitzgibbons, R.P. (2000). *Helping Clients Forgive: An Empirical Guide for Resolving Anger and Restoring Hope.* American Psychological Association.

Enright, R.D. and Fitzgibbons, R.P. (2015). *Forgiveness Therapy.* American Psychological Association.

Ermer, A.E. and Proulx, C.M. (2016). Unforgiveness, depression, and health in later life: the protective factor of forgivingness. *Aging & Mental Health* 20(10): 1021–1034. https://doi.org/10.1080/13607863.2015.1060942.

Eurich, T. (2017). *Insight.* Macmillan.

Farkas, C.M. and Wetlaufer, S. (1996). The way chief executive officers lead. *Harvard Business Review* 74(3): 110–122.

Fletcher, C. and Bailey, C. (2003). Assessing self-awareness: some issues and methods. *Journal of Managerial Psychology* 18(5): 395–404. https://doi.org/10.1108/02683940310484008.

Frone, M.R. (2016). Work stress and alcohol use: developing and testing a biphasic self-medication model. *Work and Stress* 30(4): 374–394. https://doi.org/10.1080/02678373.2016.1252971.

Gagnier, J.J., Kienle, G., Altman, D.G. et al. (2012). The CARE guidelines: consensus-based clinical case reporting guideline development. *Global Advances in Health and Medicine* 2(5): 38–43. https://doi.org/10.7453/gahmj.2012.1.1.001.

Gallagher, C.T., Attopley, M., Gossel, T. et al. (2022). Fitness-to-practice determinations after academic dishonesty among health professions in the United Kingdom. *Journal of Nursing Regulation* 13(1): 54–61. https://doi.org/10.1016/S2155-8256(22)00034-5.

Gascon, M., Zijlema, W., Vert, C. et al. (2017). Outdoor blue spaces, human health and well-being: a systematic review of quantitative studies. *International Journal of Hygiene and Environmental Health* 220(8): 1207–1221. https://doi.org/10.1016/j.ijheh.2017.08.004.

Gelbart, N.R. (1998). *The King's Midwife: A History and Mystery of Madame du Coudray.* University of California Press.

Gerada, C. (2021). *Beneath the White Coat: Doctors, Their Minds and Mental Health.* Routledge.

Germer, C.K. and Neff, K.D. (2013). Self compassion in clinical practice. *Journal of Clinical Psychology* 69(8): 856–867.

Giffard, W. (1734). *Cases in Midwifery [sic].* Revised and Published by (ed. B. Motte, T. Wotton, and L. Gilliver).

Gismero-González, E., Jódar, R., Martínez, M.P. et al. (2020). Interpersonal offenses and psychological well-being: the mediating role of forgiveness. *Journal of Happiness Studies* 21(1): 75–94. https://doi.org/10.1007/s10902-018-00070-x.

Godbole, P. (2017). Why do people resist change? In: *Why Hospitals Fail* (ed. P. Godbole, D. Burke, and J. Aylott), 149–156. Springer International Publishing https://doi.org/10.1007/978-3-319-56224-7_15.

Goffman, E. (1959). *The Presentation of Self in Everyday Life.* Doubleday.

Goleman, D. (1996). Emotional intelligence: why it can matter more than IQ. *Learning* 24(6): 49–50.

Goman, C. (2020). *Stand Out: How to Build Your Leadership Presence.* Kogan Page.

Goodman, D., Ogrinc, G., Davies, L. et al. (2016). Explanation and elaboration of the SQUIRE (standards for quality improvement reporting excellence) guidelines, V.2.0: examples of SQUIRE elements in the healthcare improvement literature. *BMJ Quality and Safety* 25(12): e7. https://doi.org/10.1136/bmjqs-2015-004480.

Green, B., Oeppen, R.S., Smith, D.W., and Brennan, P.A. (2017). Challenging hierarchy in healthcare teams – ways to flatten gradients to improve teamwork and patient care. *British Journal of Oral and Maxillofacial Surgery* 55(5): 449–453. https://doi.org/10.1016/j.bjoms.2017.02.010.

Griffiths, R. (2004). Knowledge production and the research–teaching nexus: the case of the built environment disciplines. *Studies in Higher Education* 29(6): 709–726. https://doi.org/10.1080/0307507042000287212.

Grundy, I. (1995). Sarah stone: enlightenment midwife. In: *Medicine in the Enlightment*, 128–144. Brill.

Habibzadeh, F. and Yadollahie, M. (2010). Are shorter article titles more attractive for citations? Cross-sectional study of 22 scientific journals. *Croatian Medical Journal* 51(2): 165–170. https://doi.org/10.3325/cmj.2010.51.165.

Hagley, G., Mills, P.D., Watts, B.V., and Wu, A.W. (2019). Review of alternatives to root cause analysis: developing a robust system for incident report analysis. *BMJ Open Quality* 8(3): e000646. https://doi.org/10.1136/bmjoq-2019-000646.

Hankivsky, O. (2014). *Intersectionality 101*. The Institute for Intersectionality Research and Policy.

Harel, Z., Silver, S.A., McQuillan, R.F. et al. (2016). How to diagnose solutions to a quality of care problem. *Clinical Journal of the American Society of Nephrology* 11(5): 901–907. https://doi.org/10.2215/CJN.11481015.

Harrington, J.M. (2001). Health effects of shift work and extended hours of work. *Occupational and Environmental Medicine* 58(1): 68–72. https://doi.org/10.1136/oem.58.1.68.

Harris, J., Newton, M., Dawson, K., and Sandall, J. (2019). Implementation science in maternity care. In: *Squaring the Circle: Researching Normal Birth in a Technological World* (ed. S. Downe and S. Byrom), 253–268. Pinter and Martin.

Haxby, E. and Shuldham, C. (2018). How to undertake a root cause analysis investigation to improve patient safety. *Nursing Standard* 32(20): 41–46.

Healey, M. (2005). Linking research and teaching to benefit student learning. *Journal of Geography in Higher Education* 29(2): 183–201. https://doi.org/10.1080/03098260500130387.

Health and Safety Executive (2019). *Tackling Work-Related Stress Using the Management Standards Approach: A Step-by-Step Workbook*. The Stationery Office.

Heinrichs, M., Baumgartner, T., Kirschbaum, C., and Ehlert, U. (2003). Social support and oxytocin interact to suppress cortisol and subjective responses to psychosocial stress. *Biological Psychiatry* 54: 1389–1398.

Homer, C.S.E., Friberg, I.K., Dias, M.A.B. et al. (2014). The projected effect of scaling up midwifery. *The Lancet* 384(9948): 1146–1157. https://doi.org/10.1016/S0140-6736(14)60790-X.

ten Hoope-Bender, P. and Renfrew, M.J. (2014). Midwifery – a vital path to quality maternal and newborn care: the story of the Lancet Series on Midwifery. *Midwifery* 30(11): 1105–1106. https://doi.org/10.1016/j.midw.2014.08.010.

Howell, E.A., Sofaer, S., Balbierz, A. et al. (2022). Distinguishing high-performing from low-performing hospitals for severe maternal morbidity: a focus on quality and equity. *Obstetrics and Gynaecology* 139(6): 1061.

Hunter, B., Fenwick, J., Sidebotham, D.M., and Henley, D.J. (2019). Midwives in the United Kingdom: levels of burnout, depression, anxiety and stress and associated predictors. *Midwifery* 79. https://doi.org/10.1016/j.midw.2019.08.008.

Husereau, D., Drummond, M., Petrou, S. et al. (2013). Consolidated health economic evaluation reporting standards (cheers) statement. *International Journal of Technology Assessment in Health Care* 29(2): 117–122. https://doi.org/10.1017/S0266462313000160.

Ibarra, H. and Hunter, M. (2007). How leaders create and use networks. *Harvard Business Review,* 35(1).

Jackson, E.M. (2013). STRESS RELIEF: the role of exercise in stress management. *ACSM's Health & Fitness Journal* 17(3): 14–19. https://doi.org/10.1249/FIT.0b23e31828cb1c9.

Jones, A., Neal, A., Bailey, S., and Cooper, A. (2023). When work harms: how better understanding of avoidable employee harm can improve employee safety, patient safety and healthcare quality. *BMJ Leader.* https://doi.org/10.1136/leader-2023-000849.

Jones-Berry, S. (2016). Suicide risk for nurses during fitness to practise process: staff investigated by nursing regulator say they experience stress, long delays and too little communication. *Mental Health Practice* 19(8): 8–9. https://doi.org/10.7748/mhp.19.8.8.s9.

Jung, C. (1973). *Letters*, vol. 1, 1906–1950. Princeton University Press.

Kahneman, D., Lovallo, D., and Sibony, O. (2011). Before you make that big decision. *Harvard Business Review* 89(6): 50–60.

Katou, A.A. and Budhwar, P.S. (2010). Causal relationship between HRM policies and organisational performance: evidence from the Greek manufacturing sector. *European Management Journal* 28(1): 25–39. https://doi.org/10.1016/j.emj.2009.06.001.

Kinman, G., Teoh, K., and Harris, A. (2020). *Mental Health and Wellbeing of Nurses and Midwives in the UK.* https://eprints.bbk.ac.uk/policies.html

Kline, R. and Lewis, D. (2019). The price of fear: estimating the financial cost of bullying and harassment to the NHS in England. *Public Money & Management* 39(3): 166–174. https://doi.org/10.1080/09540962.2018.1535044.

Kneafsey, R., Brown, S., Sein, K. et al. (2016). A qualitative study of key stakeholders' perspectives on compassion in healthcare and the development of a framework for compassionate interpersonal relations. *Journal of Clinical Nursing* 25(1–2): 70–79. https://doi.org/10.1111/jocn.12964.

Konstam, V., Chernoff, M., and Deveney, S. (2001). Toward forgiveness: the role of shame, guilt anger, and empathy. *Counseling and Values* 46(1): 26–39. https://doi.org/10.1002/j.2161-007X.2001.tb00204.x.

Kotter, J.P. and Schlesinger, L.A. (1989). *Choosing Strategies for Change.* Macmillan Education UK.

Lazarus, R.S. and Folkman, S. (1991). The concept of coping. In: *Stress and Coping: An Anthology* (ed. A. Monat and R.S. Lazarus), 189–206. Columbia University Press.

Lee, E.E., Govind, T., Ramsey, M. et al. (2021). Compassion toward others and self-compassion predict mental and physical well-being: a 5-year longitudinal study of 1090 community-dwelling adults across the lifespan. *Translational Psychiatry* 11(1): 397. https://doi.org/10.1038/s41398-021-01491-8.

Liberati, E.G., Tarrant, C., Willars, J. et al. (2021). Seven features of safety in maternity units: a framework based on multisite ethnography and stakeholder consultation. *BMJ Quality and Safety* 30(6): 444–456. https://doi.org/10.1136/bmjqs-2020-010988.

Loi, N., Golledge, C., and Schutte, N. (2021). Negative affect as a mediator of the relationship between emotional intelligence and uncivil workplace behaviour among managers. *Journal of Management Development* 40(1): 94–103. https://doi.org/10.1108/JMD-12-2018-0370.

Luc, J., Archer, M., Arora, R. et al. (2021). Does tweeting improve citations? One-year results from the TSSMN prospective randomised trial. *The Annals of Thoracic Surgery* 111 (1): 296–300.

Lugones, M. (2010). Toward a decolonial feminism. *Hypatia* 25(4): 742–759. https://doi.org/10.1111/j.1527-2001.2010.01137.x.

Lundgren, T., Luoma, J.B., Dahl, J. et al. (2012). The bull's-eye values survey: a psychometric evaluation. *Cognitive and Behavioral Practice* 19(4): 518–526. https://doi.org/10.1016/j.cbpra.2012.01.004.

Maben, J., Taylor, C., Reynolds, E. et al. (2021). Realist evaluation of Schwartz rounds® for enhancing the delivery of compassionate healthcare: understanding how they work, for whom, and in what contexts. *BMC Health Services Research* 21(1): 709. https://doi.org/10.1186/s12913-021-06483-4.

Maben, J., Conolly, A., Abrams, R. et al. (2022). 'You can't walk through water without getting wet' UK nurses' distress and psychological health needs during the Covid-19 pandemic: a longitudinal interview study. *International Journal of Nursing Studies* 131: 104242. https://doi.org/10.1016/j.ijnurstu.2022.104242.

Maben, J., Taylor, C., Jagosh, J. et al. (2023). *Delivering Healthcare: A Complex Balancing Act: A Guide to Understanding Psychological Ill-Health in Nurses, Midwives and Paramedics.* University of Surrey.

Majid, U. and Vanstone, M. (2018). Appraising qualitative research for evidence syntheses: a compendium of quality appraisal tools. *Qualitative Health Research* 28(13): 2115–2131. https://doi.org/10.1177/1049732318785358.

Mancl, A.C. and Penington, B. (2011). Tall poppies in the workplace: communication strategies used by envious others in response to successful women. *Qualitative Research Reports in Communication* 12(1): 79–86. https://doi.org/10.1080/17459435.2011.601701.

Marland, H. (1993). *The Art of Midwifery: Early Modern Midwives in Europe.* Routledge.

Matheson, K. and Anisman, H. (2003). Systems of coping with dysphoria, anxiety and depressive illness: a multivariate profile perspective. *Stress* 6: 223–234.

McKenna, H. (1991). The developments and trends in relation to men practising midwifery: a review of the literature. *Journal of Advanced Nursing* 16(4): 480–489.

Merlo, L.J., Campbell, M.D., Shea, C. et al. (2022). Essential components of physician health program monitoring for substance use disorder: a survey of participants 5 years post successful program completion. *The American Journal on Addictions* 31(2): 115–122. https://doi.org/10.1111/ajad.13257.

Moher, D., Liberati, A., Tetzlaff, J., and Altman, D.G. (2009). Preferred reporting items for systematic reviews and meta-analyses: the PRISMA statement. *Annals of Internal Medicine* 151(4): 336–341.

Morgensen, S.L. (2011). The biopolitics of settler colonialism: right here, right now. *Settler Colonial Studies* 1(1): 52–76. https://doi.org/10.1080/2201473X.2011.10648801.

Morgensen, S.L. (2012). Theorising gender, sexuality and settler colonialism: an introduction. *Settler Colonial Studies* 2(2): 2–22. https://doi.org/10.1080/2201473X.2012.10648839.

Morison, T. (2021). Reproductive justice: a radical framework for researching sexual and reproductive issues in psychology. *Social and Personality Psychology Compass* 15(6): https://doi.org/10.1111/spc3.12605.

Morris, Z.S., Wooding, S., and Grant, J. (2011). The answer is 17 years, what is the question: understanding time lags in translational research. *Journal of the Royal Society of Medicine* 104: 510–520.

Neff, K. (2003a). Self-compassion: an alternative conceptualization of a healthy attitude toward oneself. *Self and Identity* 2(2): 85–101. https://doi.org/10.1080/15298860309032.

Neff, K.D. (2003b). The development and validation of a scale to measure self-compassion. *Self and Identity* 2(3): 223–250. https://doi.org/10.1080/15298860309027.

Neff, K.D. and Knox, M.C. (2017). Self-compassion. In: *Encyclopedia of Personality and Individual Differences* (ed. V. Zeigler-Hill and T.K. Shackelford), 1–8. Springer International Publishing. https://doi.org/10.1007/978-3-319-28099-8_1159-1.

Newman, A., Donohue, R., and Eva, N. (2017). Psychological safety: a systematic review of the literature. *Human Resource Management Review* 27(3): 521–535. https://doi.org/10.1016/j.hrmr.2017.01.001.

Ng, L., Schache, K., Young, M., and Sinclair, J. (2023). Value of Schwartz rounds in promoting the emotional well-being of healthcare workers: a qualitative study. *BMJ Open* 13(4): e064144. https://doi.org/10.1136/bmjopen-2022-064144.

NMC (2019). Nursing and Midwifery Council Register. Nursing and Midwifery Council. www.nmc.org.uk

Nove, A., ten Hoope-Bender, P., Boyce, M. et al. (2021). The state of the world's midwifery 2021 report: findings to drive global policy and practice. *Human Resources for Health* 19(1): 146. https://doi.org/10.1186/s12960-021-00694-w.

O'Brien, B.C., Ilene, B.H., Thomas, J.B. et al. (2014). Standards for reporting qualitative research: a synthesis of recommendations. *Academic Medicine* 89(9): 1245–1251.

Ockenden, D. (2022). *Ockenden Report – Final: Return to an Address of the Honourable the House of Commons dated 30 March 2022 for Findings, Conclusions and Essential Actions from the Independent Review of Maternity Services at the Shrewsbury and Telford Hospital NHS Trust: Our Final Report*. Dandy Booksellers Ltd.

O'Sullivan, S. (2021). The colonial project of gender (and everything else). *Genealogy* 5(3): 67. https://doi.org/10.3390/genealogy5030067.

Page, M.J., McKenzie, J.E., and Higgins, J.P.T. (2018). Tools for assessing risk of reporting biases in studies and syntheses of studies: a systematic review. *BMJ Open* 8(3): e019703. https://doi.org/10.1136/bmjopen-2017-019703.

Pearce, G., Bell, L., Pezaro, S., and Reinhold, E. (2023a). Childbearing with hypermobile Ehlers–Danlos syndrome and hypermobility spectrum disorders: a large international survey of outcomes and complications. *International Journal of Environmental Research and Public Health* 20(20): 6957. https://doi.org/10.3390/ijerph20206957.

Pearce, G., Bell, L., Magee, P., and Pezaro, S. (2023b). Co-created solutions for perinatal professionals and childbearing needs for people with hypermobile Ehlers-Danlos syndrome and hypermobility spectrum disorders. *International Journal of Environmental Research and Public Health* 20(20): 6955. https://doi.org/10.3390/ijerph20206955.

Peeters, B. (2004). Tall poppies and egalitarianism in Australian discourse: from key word to cultural value. *English World-Wide. A Journal of Varieties of English* 25(1): 1–25. https://doi.org/10.1075/eww.25.1.02pee.

Pendleton, J. (2019). What role does gender have in shaping knowledge that underpins the practice of midwifery? *Journal of Gender Studies* 28(6): 629–634. https://doi.org/10.1080/09589236.2019.1590185.

Pennebaker, J.W. (1997). Writing about emotional experiences as a therapeutic process. *Psychological Science* 8(3): 162–166. https://doi.org/10.1111/j.1467-9280.1997.tb00403.x.

Pezaro, S. (2019). Midwives in 2020: time to flourish and change perceptions. *British Journal of Midwifery* 27(12): 746–747.

Pezaro, S., Clyne, W., Turner, A. et al. (2016). 'Midwives Overboard!' Inside their hearts are breaking, their makeup may be flaking but their smile still stays on. *Women and Birth* 29(3): e59–e66. https://doi.org/10.1016/j.wombi.2015.10.006.

Pezaro, S., Clyne, W., and Fulton, E.A. (2017). A systematic mixed-methods review of interventions, outcomes and experiences for midwives and student midwives in work-related psychological distress. *Midwifery* 50: 163–173. https://doi.org/10.1016/j.midw.2017.04.003.

Pezaro, S., Pearce, G., and Bailey, E. (2018a). Childbearing women's experiences of mid-wives' workplace distress: patient and public involvement. *British Journal of Midwifery* 26(10): 659–669. https://doi.org/10.12968/bjom.2018.26.10.659.

Pezaro, S., Pearce, G., and Reinhold, E. (2018b). Hypermobile Ehlers-Danlos syndrome during pregnancy, birth and beyond. *British Journal of Midwifery* 26(4): 217–223. https://doi.org/10.12968/bjom.2018.26.4.217.

Pezaro, D.S., Pearce, D.G., and Reinhold, D.E. (2020a). Understanding hypermobile Ehlers-Danlos syndrome and hypermobility spectrum disorders in the context of childbearing: an international qualitative study. *Midwifery* 88: 102749. https://doi.org/10.1016/j.midw.2020.102749.

Pezaro, S., Patterson, J., Moncrieff, G., and Ghai, I. (2020b). A systematic integrative review of the literature on midwives and student midwives engaged in problematic substance use. *Midwifery* 89: 102785. https://doi.org/10.1016/j.midw.2020.102785.

Pezaro, S., Maher, K., Bailey, E., and Pearce, G. (2021a). Problematic substance use: an assessment of workplace implications in midwifery. *Occupational Medicine (Oxford, England)* 71(9): 460–466. https://doi.org/10.1093/occmed/kqab127.

Pezaro, S., Pearce, G., and Reinhold, E. (2021b). A clinical update on hypermobile Ehlers-Danlos syndrome during pregnancy, birth and beyond. *British Journal of Midwifery* 29(9): 492–500. https://doi.org/10.12968/bjom.2021.29.9.492.

Pezaro, S., Jenkins, M., and Bollard, M. (2022a). Defining 'research inspired teaching' and introducing a research inspired online/offline teaching (RIOT) framework for fostering it using a co-creation approach. *Nursing Education Today* 108: 105–163.

Pezaro, S., Maher, K., Bailey, E., and Pearce, G. (2022b). Problematic substance use in midwives registered with the United Kingdom's Nursing and Midwifery Council: a pragmatic mixed methods study. *Midwifery* 103409. https://doi.org/10.1016/j.midw.2022.103409.

Pezaro, S., Maher, K., and Fissell, M. (2022c). Midwives need a useable past to shape their future. *The Lancet* 399(10329): 1046–1047. https://doi.org/10.1016/S0140-6736(22)00231-8.

Pezaro, S., Crowther, R., Pearce, G. et al. (2023). Perinatal care for trans and nonbi-nary people birthing in heteronormative "maternity" services: experiences and educational needs of professionals. *Gender & Society* 37(1): 124–151. https://doi.org/10.1177/08912432221138086.

Popper, K. (1959). *The Logic of Scientific Discovery*. Routledge Classics.

Porritt, K., Gomersall, J., and Lockwood, C. (2014). Study selection and critical appraisal. *American Journal of Nursing* 114(6): 47–52.

Prescott-Clements, L., Voller, V., Bell, M. et al. (2017). Rethinking remediation: a model to support the detailed diagnosis of clinicians' performance problems and the development of effective remediation plans. *Journal of Continuing Education in the Health Professions* 37(4): 245–254. https://doi.org/10.1097/CEH.0000000000000173.

Price, T., Wong, G., Withers, L. et al. (2021). Optimising the delivery of remediation programmes for doctors: a realist review. *Medical Education* 55(9): 995–1010. https://doi.org/10.1111/medu.14528.

Rayner, C., Hoel, H., and Cooper, C. (2002). *Workplace Bullying: What We Know, Who Is to Blame and What We Can Do?* Taylor and Francis.

Roter, A. (2018). *The Dark Side of the Workplace: Managing Incivility*. Routledge.

Royal College of Midwives (2017). *The Gathering Storm: Englands Midwifery Workforce Challenges*. Royal College of Midwives.

Royal College of Obstetricians and Gynaecologists (2020). *Each Baby Counts: 2020 Final Progress Report*. Royal College of Obstetricians and Gynaecologists.

Salas, E., Sims, D.E., and Burke, C.S. (2005). Is there a "big five" in teamwork? *Small Group Research* 36(5): 555–599. https://doi.org/10.1177/1046496405277134.

Sannomiya, M., Sasagawa, E., Hikita, N. et al. (2019). The proportions, regulations, and training plans of male midwives worldwide: a descriptive study of 77 countries. *International Journal of Childbirth* 9(1): 5–18. https://doi.org/10.1891/2156-5287.9.1.5.

Schulz, K.F., Altman, D.G., and Moher, D. (2010). CONSORT 2010 statement: updated guidelines for reporting parallel group randomised trials. *Journal of Pharmacology and Pharmacotherapeutics* 1(2): 100–107.

Serrat, O. (2017). The five whys technique. In: *Knowledge Solutions* (ed. O. Serrat), 307–310. Singapore: Springer https://doi.org/10.1007/978-981-10-0983-9_32.

Shiffer, D., Minonzio, M., Dipaola, F. et al. (2018). Effects of clockwise and counterclockwise job shift work rotation on sleep and work-life balance on hospital nurses. *International Journal of Environmental Research and Public Health* 15(9): 2038. https://doi.org/10.3390/ijerph15092038.

Sidhu, D.S. (2020). Criminal law x addiction. *NCL Rev* 99: 1083.

Silvia, P.J. and O'Brien, M.E. (2004). Self-awareness and constructive functioning: revisiting "the Human Dilemma". *Journal of Social and Clinical Psychology* 23(4): 475–489. https://doi.org/10.1521/jscp.23.4.475.40307.

Small, K.A., Sidebotham, M., Fenwick, J., and Gamble, J. (2022). Midwives must, obstetricians may: an ethnographic exploration of how policy documents organise intrapartum fetal monitoring practice. *Women and Birth* 35(2): e188–e197. https://doi.org/10.1016/j.wombi.2021.05.001.

Smallen, D. (2019). Practicing forgiveness: a framework for a routine forgiveness practice. *Spirituality in Clinical Practice* 6(4): 219–228. https://doi.org/10.1037/scp0000197.

Smith, L., Folkard, S., Tucker, P., and Macdonald, I. (1998). Work shift duration: a review comparing eight hour and 12 hour shift systems. *Occupational and Environmental Medicine* 55(4): 217–229. https://doi.org/10.1136/oem.55.4.217.

Speak, M. and Aitken-Swan, J. (1982). *Male Midwives: A Report of Two Studies*. Department of Health and Social Security.

Stone, S. (1737). *A Complete Practice of Midwifery*. Paternoster Row: The Globe.

Stroup DF, Berlin JA, Morton SC, et al, for the Meta-analysis Of Observational Studies in Epidemiology (MOOSE) Group. Meta-analysis of Observational Studies in Epidemiology. A Proposal for Reporting. JAMA. 2000;283(15):2008–2012. doi: 10.1001/jama.283.15.2008.

Stuewig, J., Tangney, J.P., Heigel, C. et al. (2010). Shaming, blaming, and maiming: functional links among the moral emotions, externalization of blame, and aggression. *Journal of Research in Personality* 44(1): 91–102. https://doi.org/10.1016/j.jrp.2009.12.005.

Takian, A., Sheikh, A., and Barber, N. (2012). We are bitter, but we are better off: case study of the implementation of an electronic health record system into a mental health hospital in England. *BMC Health Services Research* 12(1): 484. https://doi.org/10.1186/1472-6963-12-484.

Tatlock, L. (2005). *The Court Midwife*. University of Chicago Press.

Teoh, K., Dhensa-Khalon, R., Christensen, M. et al. (2023). *Organisational Interventions to Support Staff Wellbeing in the NHS*. Society of Occupational Medicine. www.som.org.uk/sites/som.org.uk/files/Organisational_Interventions_to_Support_Staff_Wellbeing_in_the_NHS.pdf

Tims, M., Bakker, A.B., and Derks, D. (2012). The development and validation of the Job Crafting Scale. *Journal of Vocational Behaviour* 80: 173–186.

Tong, A., Sainsbury, P., and Craig, J. (2007). Consolidated criteria for reporting qualitative research (COREQ): a 32-item checklist for interviews and focus groups. *International Journal for Quality in Health Care* 19(6): 349–357. https://doi.org/10.1093/intqhc/mzm042.

Travers, C.J. (2022). *Reflective Goal Setting: An Applied Approach to Personal and Leadership Development*. Palgrave Macmillan.

Travers, C.J., Morisano, D., and Locke, E.A. (2014). Self-reflection, growth goals, and academic outcomes: a qualitative study. *British Journal of Educational Psychology* 85: 224–241.

Uhl-Bien, M. and Marion, R. (2009). Complexity leadership in bureaucratic forms of organizing: a meso model. *The Leadership Quarterly* 20(4): 631–650. https://doi.org/10.1016/j.leaqua.2009.04.007.

United Nations (2015). A/RES/70/1 Transforming Our World: The 2030 Agenda for Sustainable Development.

Von Elm, E., Altman, D.G., Egger, M. et al. (2014). The Strengthening the Reporting of Observational Studies in Epidemiology (STROBE) statement: guidelines for reporting observational studies. *International Journal of Surgery* 12(12): 1495–1499. https://doi.org/10.1016/j.ijsu.2014.07.013.

Wadsworth, M.E. (2015). Development of maladaptive coping: a functional adaptation to chronic, uncontrollable stress. *Child Development Perspectives* 9(2): 96–100. https://doi.org/10.1111/cdep.12112.

Weller, J. (2012). Shedding new light on tribalism in health care: commentaries. *Medical Education* 46(2): 134–136. https://doi.org/10.1111/j.1365-2923.2011.04178.x.

West, M.A. (2021). *Compassionate Leadership: Sustaining Wisdom, Humanity, and Presence in Health and Social Care*. Swirling Leaf Press.

Wexley, K.N., Alexander, R.A., Greenawalt, J.P., and Couch, M.A. (1980). Attitudinal congruence and similarity as related to interpersonal evaluations in manager-subordinate dyads. *The Academy of Management Journal* 23(2): 320–330.

Williams, C. (1992). The glass escalator: hidden advantages for men in the 'female' professions. *Social Problems* 39: 253–267.

Wilson, A. (1995). *The Making of Man-Midwifery*. Harvard University Press.

Woods, R. and Galley, C. (2014). *Mrs Stone and Dr Smellie: Eighteenth-century Midwives and Their Patients*. Liverpool University Press.

Woodyatt, L. and Wenzel, M. (2019). The psychology of self-forgiveness. In: *Handbook of Forgiveness*. Routledge.

World Health Organisation (2015). European Strategic Directions for Strengthening Nursing and Midwifery Towards Health 2020 Goals.

World Health Organisation (2020). WHO Guidelines on Physical Activity and Sedentary Behavior.

World Health Organisation (2022a). Mental Health. https://www.who.int/news-room/fact-sheets/detail/mental-health-strengthening-our-response

World Health Organisation (2022b). Strengthening Primary Health Care to Tackle Racial Discrimination.

World Health Organization (2019). Delivered by Women, Led by Men: A Gender and Equity Analysis of the Global Health and Social Workforce. https://apps.who.int/iris/handle/10665/311322

Wrzesniewski, A. and Dutton, J.E. (2001). Crafting a job: revisioning employees as active crafters of their work. *Academy of Management Review* 26(2): 179–201.

Yoong, W., Patra-Das, S., Jeffers, N. et al. (2021). Developing situational awareness ('helicopter view'). *The Obstetrician & Gynaecologist* 23(1): 60–66. https://doi.org/10.1111/tog.12709.

Yukl, G. (2013). *Power in Organisations*. Pearson.

Index

Note: Page numbers followed by an "f" denote figures; those followed by a "t" denote tables.

Surviving and Thriving in Midwifery, First Edition. Sally Pezaro and Karen Maher.
© 2025 John Wiley & Sons Ltd. Published 2025 by John Wiley & Sons Ltd.

Printed and bound by CPI Group (UK) Ltd, Croydon, CR0 4YY

14/04/2025

14657309-0001